THE PERFECT HUMAN DIET™

"A POWERFUL documentary with scientific focus, the movie got its audience talking about what they should be eating for optimal health. As they left the theater conversations could be heard on the subject of the paleo diet and animal protein's central role in human evolution"
—**Jeremy Russell**, North American Meat Association Communications

"A recent food documentary... may be the last and only one you will ever need to watch."
—**Andrew Frezza**, Living SuperHuman

"THANK YOU for making this film. I am an anthropology as well as a nutrition nut and the prospect of a film that intelligently combines the two is very, very exciting... Can't wait to own my copy."
—**Rebecca**, Prod. Circle Film supporter

"CJ Hunt has created something INCREDIBLY VALUABLE here. Acknowledging the often conflicting and confusing health dictates of the media, *The Perfect Human Diet* leads us through the often emotional and frequently special interest-generated quagmire toward what is truly the "perfect human diet" by taking the viewer home to our most fundamental roots as a species. Through reviewing our anthropological history, scholarly insights and the irrefutable evidence of scientific isotopic analysis he brings us to an inescapable conclusion: Regardless of ideology or ethnicity we are ALL hunter-gatherers."
—**Nora Gedgaudas**, CNS, CNT

"I recently had the opportunity to see C. J. Hunt's documentary, *The Perfect Human Diet,* and I can tell you that this is going to make waves. He's done a FANTASTIC piece of investigative journalism leaves no doubt about which diet is the best match for the human genome. This is the scientific evidence that the world, especially the media, needs to see in order to find solutions for the epidemic of obesity and chronic diseases that threaten our well-being and our very survival, both individually and as a society."
—**Judy Barnes Baker,** Cookbook Author, Artist, and Writer

THE PERFECT
HUMAN DIET™

*THE SIMPLE DOCTOR-PROVEN SOLUTION FOR THE
HEALTH AND LIFE YOU DESERVE*

C.J. HUNT

New York

THE PERFECT HUMAN DIET™

THE SIMPLE DOCTOR-PROVEN SOLUTION FOR THE HEALTH AND LIFE YOU DESERVE

© 2016 **C.J. HUNT**.

Published in New York, New York, by Morgan James Publishing. Morgan James and The Entrepreneurial Publisher are trademarks of Morgan James, LLC.
www.MorganJamesPublishing.com

The Morgan James Speakers Group can bring authors to your live event. For more information or to book an event visit The Morgan James Speakers Group at www.TheMorganJamesSpeakersGroup.com.

Disclaimer: This book and the views and statements expressed in this book are not intended to be a substitute for professional medical advice. Readers should always seek their own professional advice for any medical condition, or if they think they may have a medical emergency. Readers should exercise their own care skill and diligence with respect to the reliance and use of any information contained in the book, and should not act or refrain from acting on the basis of the views and statements expressed in the book without first taking appropriate professional advice regarding their own particular circumstances.

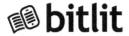

A free eBook edition is available with the purchase of this print book.

CLEARLY PRINT YOUR NAME ABOVE IN UPPER CASE

Instructions to claim your free eBook edition:
1. Download the BitLit app for Android or iOS
2. Write your name in **UPPER CASE** on the line
3. Use the BitLit app to submit a photo
4. Download your eBook to any device

ISBN 978-1-63047-544-4 paperback
ISBN 978-1-63047-545-1 eBook
ISBN 978-1-63047-546-8 hardcover
Library of Congress Control Number:
2014959976

Cover Design by:
Chris Treccani
www.3dogdesign.net

In an effort to support local communities and raise awareness and funds, Morgan James Publishing donates a percentage of all book sales for the life of each book to Habitat for Humanity Peninsula and Greater Williamsburg.

Get involved today, visit
www.MorganJamesBuilds.com

Habitat
for Humanity®
Peninsula and
Greater Williamsburg
Building Partner

TABLE OF CONTENTS

A NEW BEGINNING

At 9:05am on a hot, smoggy Memorial Day in 1978 I went jogging with a friend at Beverly Hills High School. A lap and a half later, I dropped dead of a cardiac arrest.

As I regained consciousness, I couldn't breathe. Thankfully, the emergency plastic breathing tube was pulled out of my throat and air quickly rushed in. I heard my friend Stan somewhere in the distance saying *CJ! You had a heart attack!* Followed by vague impressions of other voices as I felt myself lifted into the ambulance. Doors slammed. Sirens screamed. It was 9:38am, 20-minutes since I hit the ground. I was 24 years old.

A few days later, diagnosed with a severe heart birth defect, I could see those frightening minutes had given me another chance to live. Beginning a journey to learn how to live my healthiest life.

Now, 37 years later, even with the new challenges of a worsening heart condition and defibrillator implant, I have been able to achieve my dream to contribute something positive to life. That, as you may already know, is my investigative documentary, *The Perfect Human Diet*. The film shares my journalistic search for the solution to our epidemic of obesity and diet-related disease—the #1 killer in the U.S—and explores the unexpected answer to these problems: scientific proof of the authentic human diet.

My sincerest dream now is that the surprising and previously unknowable discoveries from my search, first revealed in the film and now in this book, will help empower you to take control of your own health where you can, creating the health and life you deserve.

Preface
FROM REPORTER TO ADVOCATE

I never intended to become an advocate for these new scientific discoveries. When I began my search for the solution to diet-related obesity and chronic disease, my journalistic goal with my film *The Perfect Human Diet* was to remain solely an objective reporter. I planned to let the film's researchers and scientific experts speak to their latest discoveries in the newly emerging field of "human evolutionary nutrition," keeping my own opinions to myself. The hard scientific evidence would stand on its own, whatever I found. This way, my investigative documentary, whose creation was inspired by the late ABC News Anchor Peter Jennings' "*In Search of…*" TV specials, and the early journalistic curiosity of Phil Donahue and Oprah Winfrey on their talk shows, wouldn't be an intentional sales piece produced in an effort to convince you that "I'm right," and that you should live the way I advise. As a viewer, you watch the film, and then decide for yourself if and how you want to utilize the film's discoveries to optimize your health.

So what inspired this new direction of advocacy? Unexpectedly, two things happened to inspire me to take this new tact. The first occurred while I was watching the original uncut interview footage in the editing room. I was able then to focus on the interviews' content in a way that wasn't possible while conducting the interviews. It struck me that the film crew and I had recorded critical revelations about the human diet, both past and present, and its relationship to our health, that was previously unknowable. I realized that this was truly game-changing information that everyone with interest in their own health and that of their loved ones should know about.

The second thing that spurred me to advocacy was meeting with audience members over the first few months of the film's premier screenings. Many of them approached me after watching the film to ask me what *I* eat every day? Could I give them some advice, answer a few questions on making the method of eating described by Dr. Lane Sebring in the film, easy? Could I help guide them towards the kind of positive results I was experiencing, even with my heart condition? Now that they had seen the film and the film's discoveries, the result of 10-years effort and more than 35 years of my own dietary experimentation searching for optimal health (and the happiness that goes with it), they, too, wanted "first person" practical everyday ideas. They viewed me as an "expert by experience" who they could relate to. I was moved and inspired by their belief in me and by their heartfelt questions.

One woman in particular said something to me while I was in the Midwest that really hit home. A silver-haired woman in her sixties stepped up to me in the small Mississippi River town of Canton, Missouri, after traveling with her husband over 100 miles to see the film. She said that for decades she had been suffering, and continued to suffer, the same rapid fluctuations in blood sugar which I had described in the film as one of my own experiences while following a low-fat, high-carbohydrate USDA "food pyramid" (now "food plate") directed diet.[1] She told me in some detail how those fluctuations over these many years were robbing her of her vitality and enthusiasm for life. Then we chatted about the method of eating she could follow based on the discoveries of the film and Dr. Lane Sebring's medical advice to his patients. Finally, as we neared the end of our conversation and took each other's hands to say goodbye, she added, "This gives me hope that I can feel good again—I just want to feel good again." After some reflection on that moment and others like it, I decided to write this book to the see what more I can do to help people find the health and life they deserve.

---

1   In my case, those blood sugar fluctuations were diagnosed as a potentially pre-diabetic condition now widely understood as acute hypoglycemia.

To be clear, it was never my intention to write a diet book, and I still don't believe this is a diet book but rather a story of discovery, scientific innovation, history and how the authentic human diet was, and still is, the best way for us to obtain optimal health and well being. When I made the documentary *The Perfect Human Diet*, my father asked me what was different about this film, not in its content, but in its approach. I wasn't sure how to answer this as my mind was wrapped around the facts and figures of the film, but then my business partner spoke up and said, "It's his reporter's eye that makes this different. He has an objective presentation that no other diet stories have, and it can be enjoyed from many different angles, but leaves the self-discovery up to the viewer." And he was right; the film revealed many things that inspired and motivated viewers to change the way they think about food. Nevertheless, they started asking me questions and those questions needed answering, hence this companion book.

So, advocate it is. But not advocating my opinions. I'm here to help shed more light on the first person research and amazing science revealing to us what was previously unknowable, part of which is the truly game changing, hard science discovery of the authentic human diet. No more dietary theories, guesses or inventions – but instead, breakthrough scientific facts.

I'm also here to share with you the simplest way to put to use this discovery, through *The Perfect Human Diet's* "Human Food" and "Non-Human Food" guidelines. This simple distinction, backed by understanding a bit of our species' nutrition history, will put the human diet in a new context that can free you from dietary confusion once and for all. Adding this simple knowledge to your resources will set you on the course to make your best decisions about which foods will make you as healthy as you can possibly be—for the rest of your life.

Part One
THE TRUTH

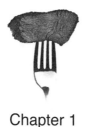

CAN YOU HANDLE THE TRUTH?

Chapter 1

"There are three things in life which are very visceral: religion, politics, and nutrition. They're all based on belief systems, and none of them respond well to challenge. Essentially we say, "Don't confuse me with the facts...because in my heart, I know I'm right."

—**Barry Sears**, PhD

How would you feel if you learned meat and healthy animal fats are irreplaceable in an optimal human diet? That the prevailing government and media message that meat and animal protein are inherently unhealthy is, simply put, wrong? That the USDA's Food Plate, along with many beloved TV and film personalities' promotion of plant based diets as the healthiest method of eating, is not based on the fullest range of available science? Would your jaw drop in disbelief? Would you be angry to learn this because, once again, you feel you were misled by politically driven misinformation or corporate self-interests that could harm you and your loved ones' health? Or perhaps, on a more personal level, because you enthusiastically invested your heart and soul into believing the recent popular message that you were born to be "plant strong," and you should be eating a plant based diet?

For years we've been told that eating animal foods and fats sets you up for coronary artery disease, cancer and a guaranteed future under the surgeons' knife. I myself tried a vegan diet for many years because I was told that was the healthiest option. If you are like I was, it's likely you struggled to eliminate animal products from your diet, change your conventional eating habits and lifestyle, even consuming low to no fat as much as possible?

Yet believe it or not, the most compelling new hard science shows that people eating animal protein and fats, the very same people you've been told repeatedly are unhealthy and headed for the operating room, are actually in sync with the authentic foundation for optimal human health *because* they eat animal protein and fats. The newest and most advanced scientific testing says it's a fact. A fact that can save and change lives. But before you get the idea this will be another in the ongoing series of attack books, rest assured, it's not. I'm a reporter and filmmaker who went on an unprecedented search in the hopes of finding a solution to the obesity epidemic and chronic diet-related disease, and during that search, was led to something completely unexpected that I am truly excited to share with you. This is why I'm taking a moment to qualify my intentions about this book. And why, at the top of the page, I featured what Barry Sears[2] said to me while I interviewed him for *The Perfect Human Diet*[3] documentary. Our very human tendency is to get really upset when something we believe in our heart must be true is challenged with different information. That includes information that's significantly upgraded, and in this case, essential for making our best health decisions.

Early in the preproduction process, I was conducting a few interview calls when I asked one physician, an advisor at that time to the president

2   Barry Sears, PhD, author of many best selling books on nutrition and health.
3   Originally titled "In Search of the Perfect Human Diet"

and CEO of the prestigious Robert Wood Johnson Foundation (RWJF), the nation's largest philanthropy dedicated solely to health and health care, if he had read *Good Calories, Bad Calories: Fats, Carbs, and the Controversial Science of Diet and Health* by science writer Gary Taubes. He replied, *"I haven't read it... and I won't read it."* Why wouldn't he read it? He said it was because he was a vegetarian, and he *"didn't want to be upset."*

That's where MY jaw dropped. Here was an M.D., advising on funding for programs to solve childhood obesity, someone who I thought would be vitally interested in scientific discovery, in upgrading his medical knowledge in order to help his patients and RWJF improve the world no matter his personal food choices—but not so. I was a bit surprised honestly. But I was to learn during the course of filming that even individuals who are highly educated, and in positions of influencing public policy and funding decisions, are not always open-minded and willing to examine their own ways of thinking. Many are still so vested in their own beliefs they are unable to be objective.

Being that I've always been inherently curious and persistent in figuring out how to fix things, this lack of professional curiosity is difficult for me to understand. This is especially surprising given that Americans are now in the middle of a terrible diet-caused health epidemic that is only getting worse, with most people confused about what to eat for optimum health. Of course, changing conventional wisdom about diet and health is a challenge. As recorded history has shown us time and time again, there is resistance on many fronts to making changes to current, conventional ways of thinking in many areas. And when it comes to what we should be eating to stay or become healthy, the authorities keep turning back to the same common dietary beliefs that have been failing, and continue, to fail us.

Why do they keep returning to the same old standards? One unsurprising, but unfortunate, reason is politics. During my search, physicians repeatedly told me that major studies funded by the U.S. and Canadian governments to research and substantiate the low-fat, low-cholesterol food recommendations did not show improved health, and in fact demonstrated the opposite. Yet, the researchers in these government-funded studies concluded that these low-fat, low-cholesterol ideas would work for us. They said, "It will just take more time." More funding. And more study to prove it's true.[4] (To this reporter it sounded a lot like the *"let's keep doing the same thing we've been doing and expect different results"* scientific method).

I was also told by the physicians and researchers who said this to me that challenging these studies was politically charged professionally. To raise your voice that there might be better science available that showed another way, another way which actually does work, could easily destroy their careers. Given the wide spread institutional support for the dietary status quo, it's not hard to believe. In spite of it seeming like a no-brainer that the personal and collective stakes are just too high now to ignore the best science available that could solve the obesity epidemic and diet related chronic disease.

Those two reasons, I believe, are a couple of the biggest issues holding us back from solving our current health crisis, at least on the national level. Another influence is too few of our political representatives can see past statistics and identify directly with the problem. Media reports often explain obesity with mind numbing statistics, graphics and projections of the huge economic costs to the country; they are impersonal and unreal. For example, in the U.S. alone, it's estimated that between three and four hundred thousand people die yearly from complications directly related to their diet. That means in the next ten years four million more American's will be dead from largely preventable causes. You'd think statistics like these would stop us in our tracks, motivate all of us, including the worlds of medicine, politics and media, to search for an immediate solution. But what dominates public policy discussions and the daily news are the same faceless numbers, ongoing reports of unsustainable health care costs and confusion about how to solve it.

To put a human face on those numbers, consider this shocking analogy. The largely preventable deaths of the three to four hundred thousand people who die in the U.S. every year, from disease caused by the diet they

---

4   Shared with author during side conversations with these experts that represent the resistance to new ideas in the scientific and nutritional communities.

eat every day, is about one hundred 9/11 World Trade Center terrorist attacks. Think about that for a moment. That is essentially the same as one 9/11 every three days - year in and year out - with no end in sight.

That horrific picture is the gut-wrenching and very personal human face on those mind numbing statistics that the public policy conversations and media coverage are missing. And unlike the instant devastation of 9/11, the effects of the dietary beliefs and practices that have created the obesity epidemic creep up on us over years. We don't have a collective national experience that changes our consciousness in an instant, opening our eyes to the very real threat to all our lives, setting the stage for an immediate universal call to action. When you put a human face on those statistics, you can easily see why it's vital that we go outside of our preconceived notions about nutrition, leaving behind the conventional beliefs that continue to fuel the epidemic.

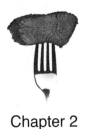

THE REAL PROBLEM DRIVING OBESITY

Chapter 2

"Americans are fat and just too confused to do anything about it."
—ABC News

For you and me, our health, our well-being, our happiness, our body, it's all very personal. We see and hear so much contradictory advice we don't really understand what to eat for optimal health. In the face of so much confusion, how can we be expected to solve a national obesity epidemic when most of us aren't even sure how to lose our own excess body fat?

Not surprisingly, this confusion over the right foods to eat for optimal health is not new. More than a decade ago a national Harris Poll found that 80% of Americans over age 25 were overweight and just *"too confused to do anything about it."* A quick Google search today on healthy eating reveals literally thousands of contradictory messages, superficial news coverage, inaccurate reporting, and personal opinions delivered as facts, fueling even more confusion. On our popular medical entertainment television shows, every day they introduce a new diet book, a new product, a new dietary supplement, a game show like demonstration, or another provocative health idea. Add to that mix our new personal media devices, like iPads, smart phones and portable computers. Escaping our confusion and uncertainty is made increasingly difficult because we are surrounded by a never-ending cycle of ever-changing diet recommendations and emotionally charged nutritional beliefs everywhere we go, every day of our lives.

It's common knowledge that in the USA low-fat, low-cholesterol, higher carbohydrate dietary beliefs have dominated the media landscape for nearly 40 years. In the last few years there has also been a significant growing bias from government, popular celebrities and medical advice television shows, who claim that plant and grain based diets are the healthiest. That said, there were a few times last year where some news and medical programs featured author-physicians whose "controversial" books brought out new evidence that commonly consumed carbohydrates elevate our blood sugar to excess, driving weight gain, diabetes and a host of inflammatory diseases, like Alzheimer's and even some cancers. As neurologist Dr. David Perlmutter said on The Dr. Oz Show recently, *"fat is back."* He continued saying, not only should we stop eating most carbohydrates we commonly consume if we want to stave off or heal Alzheimer's, but a critical component of healing and ongoing health was this: we should start eating more fats-including healthy saturated fats. In other words, we should eliminate grains and grain-based foods, sugars, most fruit, and below the ground starchy vegetables. And instead, consume more fats, such as olive oil, avocados and heart and brain healthy *saturated fats*, like butter and coconut oil. Dr. Oz, in a surprising turn around from years of conventional anti-saturated fat and anti-meat vegetarian advice actually agreed, saying, *"Heart doctors like myself, by the way, are starting to buy into this idea. Because I think you're right. What causes us to die from heart disease, and stroke, and Alzheimer's is inflammation in the body, and that's not caused by fats..."* Even though the voracious content appetite of a daily television program requires that many of the other episodes continue to promote a wide variety of dietary beliefs, a few weeks later a segment on his program again featured this new medical revelation about heart and brain healthy saturated fats, titled "The Truth about Saturated Fat."[5] Again, he agreed that new science confirms conventional wisdom claiming that saturated fats are deadly and should be avoided has been *wrong* for the last 40 years.

It's great to see television start featuring significant new scientific understandings about human nutrition, especially since animal proteins with their healthy saturated fat included solutions are still so vastly different from what has been advocated by most media for years. These kinds of breakthrough stories on television, in hindsight, will be called "defining moments" in our nutritional history. Important work from credible medical sources that should certainly help many people become much healthier as these new ideas are adopted by the general public.

Not surprisingly, while these new rays of hope come forward, there is vitriolic push back from established dietetic organizations and conventional thinking nutrition pundits rushing in to bury these new revelations in print, broadcast, and online media outlets. Again, empowering confusion.

But the good news is this: what we know about human nutrition is rapidly expanding, quickly moving away from the things we thought we knew, and the US government recommendations of the last 40 years about what foods constitute a "healthy diet." For the first time in human history, we have innovative technological advancements revealing what was previously unknowable. Some of the most extraordinary are the technologies for analyzing the archeological remains of our species. It's the moment we've been waiting for to end the dietary confusion in which we're mired.

---

5   Featuring Dr. Peter Attia, President and co-Founder with Gary Taubes of the *The Nutrition Science Initiative* (NuSI).

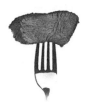

A NEW WAY OF THINKING

Chapter 3

"We can't solve problems with the same kind of thinking we used when we created them."

—Albert Einstein

"Just Tell Me What to Do" (great for book sales, not so much for you)

M ost popular diet books, the ones publishers say sell, are prescriptive plans given to us as a preset program of daily and weekly menu and recipes so we don't have to think about how to follow the diet espoused by the author. This is the *"I don't want to know why… just tell me what to do"* dieting approach that is repetitively featured on morning talk shows, selling thousands of new diet books every year. It's easy to understand that in many instances, the author's personal dietary theory, or the biology and scientific rationale of these diets, is often more complex than folks want to wrap their heads around. That's why diet book authors tell us in no uncertain terms that following their particular diet is not only the best, but incredibly easy because they've figured it all out for you. All you have to do is follow their prescription exactly, no thinking involved. It's common practice to leave the deep thinking to last year's or next year's charismatic doctor, registered dietitian or favorite celebrity author who says they have the newest ultimate solution, especially when the sales pitch is what we want to hear. We love to hear words like fast and guilt-free weight-loss plan, lose up to 18 pounds in two weeks, you can eat all the foods you love and still lose weight, eat unlimited amounts of… (insert your favorite food here).

But I'd bet in your heart-of-hearts you know that real lifetime success with any method of eating requires going a few steps further than settling, once again, for guru dependence and blindly following along. You must have your own conscious understanding of the core principles, the central idea of the diet you want to use to accomplish your goals. Then you are able to make practical choices about what to eat based on your understanding, no matter what circumstances arise.

Interestingly enough, a number of people have emailed me to say that the information the experts shared in my film made perfect sense. They finally understood the core principles, the "why" of the authentic human diet, giving them a new perspective on human nutrition. That understanding made following the film's simple guidelines easy for them, positively impacting their food choices. They passively absorbed this understanding while watching the documentary, listening to interesting stories and experts while being a part of the adventure leading to great discoveries. They found, even if it wasn't their original intention, that they had learned from this experience while being entertained. It was painless and inspired them to change their food choices—and their lives— for the better. And, they were hungry to know even more.

While the experts I spoke with explained the scientific principles and discoveries succinctly enough for the film, as you might imagine, most of our conversations could not be included, hitting the cutting room floor. So, I've taken the six most important conversations of our shared human nutrition history and included them in this book. They are presented just as they happened, written directly from the original interview transcripts. The practical application of these discoveries, the "how-two" chapters included in this companion book, use the proven strategy and unique language shared in the film that viewers found not only makes the guidelines easy to understand, but most importantly, easy to use, every day. This innovative approach also facilitates "unconscious competence"[6]; something you don't have to think about to use successfully.

The Einstein Solution — *A New Way of Thinking*

Beginning in the summer of 2006, active film production began on *The Perfect Human Diet*, an unprecedented global exploration for the solution to the obesity epidemic and diet related chronic disease. During production I had the rare opportunity to conduct on-camera interviews with an extraordinary number of researchers and scientists in multiple anthropological sciences, including unique access to the top five percent in the field of evolutionary anthropology. The vast majority of these interviews were unplanned. Special opportunities to meet with these scientists (in some truly fascinating places) that arose unexpectedly thanks to what became a common suggestion by my interviewees at the close of each interview, without my asking, *"You know who you should go talk to is…"*. In journalism and documentary filmmaking, getting the "Sure. Happy to talk to you…" for an on-camera interview, especially from scientists and researchers who don't usually give interviews, is called "unique access." It's the hoped-for opportunity when pursuing a story that most reporters and filmmakers who are not already nationally recognized can't get permission to do. And it's a great privilege when it happens. In my case, these interviews were the rare opportunity to learn from the first-person subject matter experts, the lead scientists in the

---

6   Unconscious competence: The individual has had so much refining practice with
      a skill that he or she does not really need to think about what to do. It has become
      "second nature" and can be performed with very low frequency of errors. Because
      the skill is not occupying much of the individual's conscious thoughts, it can
      often be performed while executing another task. The individual has become so
      comfortable with the skill she/he will often be able to teach it to others. http://
      en.wikipedia.org/wiki/Four_stages_of_competence

field or lab that are actually in the trenches doing the work. These were intimate conversations, demonstrations, site visits and Q&A sessions discussing the newest breakthrough information and discoveries with the best and the brightest.

For any journalist it's also exciting to have an "exclusive;" the first opportunity to share what was discussed and the revelations the conversation contained. And even more exciting to me is that these revelations, these interviews, could change the way we think about solving the obesity epidemic and diet related chronic disease; vastly improving our lives.

You may find it interesting, as I did, to know that all of these interviews were standalone conversations from a variety of scientific research specialties, and no one had prior knowledge of what any of the other experts had said to me. Yet all of the interviews pointed in the same direction, adding compelling details to the long, evolving, human nutrition story.

Many of the scientists I had this good luck to meet and interview are engaged in the emerging field of "human evolutionary nutrition." This is a particularly fascinating field of endeavor to me as they are deeply focused on discovering the secrets locked in our collective human history to advance our scientific understanding of what foods archaic and modern humans ate over time; what made us healthy, what we were eating when our health started to decline, and much more. One of the most amazing revelations I witnessed while shooting the film was seeing firsthand the newest biomolecular analysis advancements that, using hard science techniques, solve the ongoing debate about what foods constitute the authentic human diet. We can now factually define the actual food sources responsible for making us increasingly intelligent, inventive, and ultimately the planet's dominant species. No more theories, just the hard scientific facts of what was previously unknowable.

I was also directed to the first U.S. physician that fully embraced these human evolutionary nutrition principles and put them into use with his patients, with remarkable results. Everything he shared with me during filming, and our ongoing follow-up conversations about how he gets those results, is discussed in detail later in the book.

Reframing Traditional Problem Solving

When I reentered college as a mature student in my mid-40s, having previously only taken college level courses specific to journalism, I had to start as an undergraduate student at Los Angeles City College and earn my two-year AA degree, which includes many basic science courses. Then I could go on to San Francisco State University and study what I really wanted to do: television and film production with an emphasis on documentary filmmaking. Why am I telling you this? Because I learned something while in that undergraduate program that illustrates a couple of the important differences between what this book has to offer and what other books about diet offer, something that became apparent to me after the film was finished. I think you will find these distinctions will make all the difference in your ability to achieve your lifelong health goals, rather than the conventional prescription model used by popular diet books.

The New Way to Solve Problems

Early on in Psych 101 class, my professor took the time to explain how we learn and what we actually retain from our readings years after we leave school. These two new understandings were at the heart of psychology's most recent *"brain learning, memory retention, and life change research."*

1) Concepts (not prescriptions) = Behavior

He told us we all tend to forget detail rather quickly, but will remember broad concepts long after. The mind is associative[7], not linear[8], absorbing and retaining new information best when interlinking broad concepts that easily flow from one to the other. An easy way to think of this, and a

---

7   Of or relating to association, especially of ideas or images. http://www.merriam-webster.com/dictionary/associative

8   The action of laying down authoritative rules or directions. http://www.merriam-webster.com/dictionary/prescription

great image of your brain linking concepts together, is mind-mapping[9], a popular and simple tool used for brainstorming.

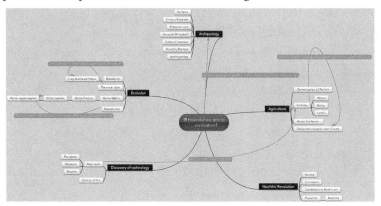

Mind Map courtesy of MindMeister www.mindmeister.com

2) Solutions by Understanding

He went on to say that that *"solutions by understanding"* are much more effective than prescriptions for life change as they create self-sufficiency in real life situations. That's great news for you and me because no matter what our social situation or circumstance, we will know what to do—or in this case, what to eat—for optimal health. This book is written with this psychological distinction in mind as a strategic reframing of traditional problem solving from solely mechanical (prescriptive), to dynamic and alive (solutions by understanding).

3) Understanding = Successful Life Change

The Perfect Human Diet guidelines presented later in this book come directly from my on-camera interviews with Dr. Lane Sebring, our enlightening "how to shop" grocery store tour (parts of which you can see in the film), and follow-up conversations with him as this companion

9   A mind map is a diagram used to visually outline information. A mind map is often created around a single word or text, placed in the center, to which associated ideas, words and concepts are added. Major categories radiate from a central node, and lesser categories are sub-branches of larger branches.[1] Categories can represent words, ideas, tasks, or other items related to a central key word or idea.(http:// en.wikipedia.org/wiki/Mind_map)

book was assembled. The doctor shared with me a completely unique, concept driven, easy to understand message and lexicon that optimizes his patients' success. No one else I met during the filming, or since, has expressed guidelines about what to eat and, just as importantly, what not to eat, in such a clear way. I'm grateful for his medical expertise. That consists of more than 15 years of direct patient experience and medical documentation. It is his wisdom that is the inspiration for this book's practical and user-friendly guide.

Think Different

Apple Inc.'s "Think Different" 1984 Super Bowl commercial[10] was a cultural game changer. An inventive play off of George Orwell's novel about totalitarianism, "1984" the commercial was set in a grey, colorless world where the population was imprisoned through the relentless universal promotion of beliefs that were to be accepted without being questioned or doubted. It focused on a brightly dressed female runner being pursued by the authorities. Escaping their grasp, she throws a sledgehammer through a giant public TV screen, smashing it and breaking through the non-stop dogma. The commercial ended heralding the coming of a new technology and a user-friendly new tool that would change our future and our lives forever: the personal computer.

Thanks to the recent advancement of innovative new scientific technologies, scientists can now answer questions about the human diet that could never be answered before. *This too is a cultural game changer.* The sledge hammer, in our case, is the hard scientific proof necessary to progress beyond thinking that the solution to our health problems lie in believing the relentless promotion of prevailing dietary recommendations.

As Einstein said, we can't solve problems with the same kind of thinking we used when we created them. And the new way of thinking we should use to solve our health and weight problems is this: "Think *Species.*"

---

10   Directed by Ridley Scott.

Part Two
THE SCIENCE

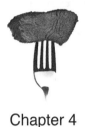

THINK SPECIES:
IT'S YOUR STORY

Chapter 4

W hen I was a boy and really wanted to know the answer to a complex question, my parents gave me straightforward and simple advice I can still hear in my memory: *"Look it up... "*. This, of course, was back in the days when we had to use books, the newspaper or a national magazine like *Life* or *Newsweek* to find answers. The Internet was many years off. *"Just think about it for a second,"* they would say to me and *"Well, Charlie, what do you think?"* Their goal was to help me become an independent thinker, stimulate my inherent drive to solve problems. Particularly, they wanted me to take the time to examine things from different angles, or different points of view, depending on whether it was a person, a place or a thing. And they always delivered their thoughts to me with a tone of encouragement.

This advice was teaching me what we now call "the pro-active approach" to finding answers. Diving in and doing our own homework. Being willing to look past conventional thinking for alternative points of view and clues. Back then if I was confused, unable to see why I couldn't get an answer or solve a problem, this is what I remember hearing the most, *"Try starting at the beginning and see where it leads you."*

Given how confused we remain about what to eat and what not to eat, starting at the beginning of our collective human story to see where it would lead was clearly the best way to get the big picture and also an objective journalistic approach to the exploration.

Species 101: *How We Got Here*

This journey through human history that I'll be sharing comes from my full interviews at the *Wenner-Gren Foundation for Anthropological Research* (New York) and other notable scientists specializing in areas of anthropology directly related to my search. Trying to wrap our minds around such a large span in time—about 2.5 million years—can make it difficult to visualize and fully understand our very personal relationship to the defining moments that 1.) made us human, and 2.) reveals the major behavioral changes that started our species down the path of a rapid decline in health.

To illustrate and simplify the time span were covering, I'll use a picture that is on a scale most of us are familiar with, a professional American football field.[11] I'll also include several screen shots from my documentary, *The Perfect Human Diet™*, so you can see things like the *American Museum of Natural History's* forensic reconstructions of what our ancestors looked liked, and the rare 2-million year old hard evidence (not on display to the public) that Physical Anthropologist Gary J. Sawyer showed me for the film.

On a completely practical level, knowing a bit more about the complete human nutrition story helps us begin to see the big picture of our human story, and following that story tells us why animal proteins and fats are essential in order for us to be as healthy as possible. Given what we've been told about diet and health most of our lives, it's also fascinating to see what has been flying under the radar of conventional

---

11 A dramatic and impactful sequence in the film also uses the football field to illustrate the journey, and clarify the reasons our species is in so much trouble with our health. For more information see www.perfecthumandiet.com

dietary beliefs, government food policy and the media's coverage of diet and health.

The Journey Begins

In the summer of 2006, I was in Leipzig, Germany, at the *Max Planck Institute for Evolutionary Anthropology* and had just concluded my interview with Professor Mick Richards, director of the Archaeological Science Group. While there, I was exposed for the first time to the remarkable technological advancements their scientists have developed that are answering questions we could never answer before about the human diet (coming in Chapter 8). The professor and I began chatting about "human evolutionary nutrition" and its direct effect on the human species in developing our large brain size. He said, *"To really understand it, you should go to the source, Professor Leslie Aiello*[12] *in New York… She's the anthropologist who wrote the paper*[13] *on how we developed big brains and small guts."*

Not long after, I was in New York with my small film crew in the offices of the Wenner-Gren Foundation about to interview Professor Leslie Aiello. I had learned while preparing for the trip that Professor Aiello's research focuses on the evolution of human adaptation, including evolution of diet, the brain, language and cognition.

Considering anthropology wasn't originally on her career radar, and taking into account her major contributions to the field, it was interesting to hear what inspired her as the camera was about to roll. As an undergrad student, Professor Aiello had had the option of taking a unique educational adventure for her summer session. In her case it was an archaeological excavation in Utah. As she told me about the trip, it was clear that she was just as excited about it now as the actual trip was to her those many years

12 Evolutionary Anthropologist and President of the *Wenner-Gren Foundation for Anthropological Research*. *The Foundation* supports significant and innovative research into humanity's biological and cultural origins, development and variation.

13 In collaboration with Peter Wheeler, she developed the Expensive Tissue Hypothesis, which posited an inverse relationship between brain size and gut size mediated through the adoption of a high quality animal-based diet. Aiello, L.C. & P. Wheeler (1995) The Expensive Tissue Hypothesis: the brain and the digestive system in human evolution. Current Anthropology 36:199 221.

ago. She said, *"I got hooked, came back from the excavation that summer, changed my major, and never looked back."*

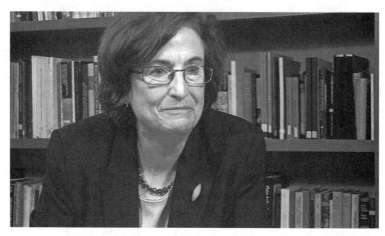

Professor Aiello started out as an "Upper[14] Paleolithic[15]" archaeologist, specializing in studying the time period around fifteen to twenty thousand years ago in Europe (The Upper Paleolithic is the third and last subdivision of the Paleolithic, which ended with the beginning of agriculture). But that soon changed, finding she was more interested in people than bones. So her interest veered to human evolution, and since the early 1970s, that has been her specialty.

The Big Picture: *Becoming Human*

The conversation that morning with Professor Aiello painted a picture about our human story I had never heard before. It was a "big picture" perspective on human evolutionary nutrition and how it resulted in our

---

14 The Upper Paleolithic (or Late Stone Age) is the third and last subdivision of the Paleolithic or Old Stone Age as it is understood in Europe, Africa and Asia. Very broadly, it dates to between 50,000 and 10,000 years ago, roughly coinciding with the appearance of behavioral modernity and before the advent of agriculture. Source: http://en.wikipedia.org/wiki/Upper_Paleolithic

15 The term "Paleolithic" was coined by archaeologist John Lubbock in 1865.[6] It derives from Greek: παλαιός, *palaios*, "old"; and λίθος, *lithos*, "stone", literally meaning "old age of the stone" or "Old Stone Age." http://en.wikipedia.org/wiki/Paleolithic

species first appearing in the African savanna, then eventually migrating out of Africa and spreading around the globe.

"What we call the ideal human diet depends on what we call human because we've had seven million years of human evolution. But throughout those seven million years we weren't human as we would define it today... For probably five million years throughout that time period, if we saw one of these ancestors on the street we'd recognize them as an ape standing on two legs, and their diet was correspondingly different. It wasn't identical to modern apes, but what we think is they were subsisting primarily upon vegetable materials; fruits, leaves, that type of thing, supplementing of course with a bit of animal material.... But at about two million years ago we think the change really happened."

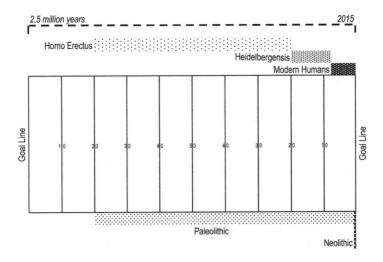

At this time our ancestors, *Homo erectus*[16], were radically different in body form from an ape standing on two legs. They were about 50

16 Early African *Homo erectus* fossils (sometimes called *Homo ergaster*) are the oldest known early humans to have possessed modern human-like body proportions with relatively elongated legs and shorter arms compared to the size of the torso. These features are considered adaptations to a life lived on the ground, indicating the loss of earlier tree-climbing adaptations, with the ability to walk and possibly

percent bigger than these earlier ancestors, and if you saw them on the street they would look more like us. They would have the same body proportions we have: long legs and relatively short arms in relation to those legs, but very importantly smaller teeth and jaws compared to those earlier ancestors.

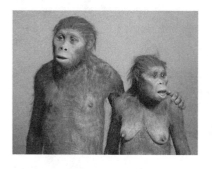 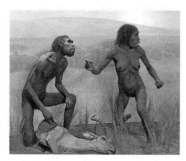

<u>*"Ape standing on two legs"*</u>

Height: Males: avg 4 ft 11 in; Females: avg 3 ft 5 in

Weight: Males: avg 92 lbs; Females: avg 64 lbs. (*Australopithecus afarensis*) http://humanorigins. si.edu/evidence/human-fossils/ species/australopithecus-afarensis

<u>*Homo erectus*</u>

Height: 4 ft 9 in - 6 ft 1 in.

Weight: 88 - 150 lbs

There was a large amount of variation in the size of *Homo erectus* individuals. The fossils from Africa indicate a larger body size than those from China, Indonesia, and the Republic of Georgia. http://humanorigins. si.edu/evidence/human-fossils/ species/homo-erectus

As Professor Aiello told me, this indicates that there was something definitely different about the diet of these ancestors at 1.7 million to 2 million years ago. The question is, what was different?

run long distances. Smithsonian Institution http://humanorigins.si.edu/evidence/human-fossils/species/homo-erectus

Animal Foods

"My own research seems to indicate that this transition involved a change to a greater proportion of animal based food. Now, this wasn't necessarily red meat because red meat is tough to chew and if you are on the African savannah you're going to be competing with a lot of other predators and you'll probably be scavenging at this time a lot of your animal based food. And the primary predators would of course go in and take out the red meat and all... What our ancestors may have been going for was the bone marrow that would give them the fats to help fuel their body; also the brains... because the predators wouldn't break into the cranial cavity, the brain cavity."

Our ancestors using rudimentary stone tools could do this. And, as I was to learn over the course of these interviews, many people in the field think that this ability was essential to get the nutrients and the long-chain fatty acids to support the evolution of the larger human brain. In fact, from the archaeological evidence, it looks like these ancestors had developed better control over acquiring animal based foods during this period. A good example, and one of the most interesting, is when you go into the archaeological sites you see the bones of these food animals. And sometimes the cut marks from the early stone tools are on the bones before the gouge marks from animal teeth. These cut marks, and the broken bones, tell us that these human ancestors were there cutting off parts of the muscle material and banging through the bones to extract marrow and brain matter before other scavengers were getting there. That's how we tell if we got there first.

"But the whole point of it is, at this stage of human evolution, the diet was changing, and we think of it as becoming much broader. Because there's also another problem. They had this bigger body size and they had to get the calories somewhere to support this large body size."

One idea many of Professor Aiello's colleagues think could work as an example of broadening the Home erectus diet is this: if those ancestors were relying more and more on rich packets of animal food that are high-energy and easy to digest, they could also then rely on some of the *"lower energy foods"* to sustain themselves. But, those would have to be the ones with bulk that contained enough carbohydrates to support this large body size. Professor Aiello asserts that the trick was to get enough extra calories from the carbohydrates *and* the fats and nutrients that would support the growth and development of the large human brain.

Big Brains, Small Guts

Something else quite interesting that has come out of Professor Aiello's work is this: we have this larger body size, and if you look at the total amount of energy we would need from our foods every day to survive, we use *exactly the same amount of energy as a mammal of our body size who has a much smaller brain.* We have these huge human brains, and brain tissue is extremely expensive in energetic terms. You might then expect that we need *more* energy because of those big brains. But we don't.

> *"I mean, depending how you measure it, our brain is about three times larger than what you would expect in an average mammal. And the mystery is, where is this energy coming from? And there is a very interesting relationship that explains this because, in comparison to the average primate (not the average mammal this time), we have very much smaller guts, smaller intestines. And if you look at the energetic costs of brain material versus your guts it's about the same. So as the bottom line, what we get in our brains we lose in our guts... and this balances our energy budget."*

To me this is one of the fascinating things about the story of our becoming human and how it relates to the changes in our diet. Remember that these particular ancestors, Homo erectus, appear in the fossil record with a new and different body form. Another distinction is that their whole chest region and down into their hips is narrower. This reason, along with the increase in brain size and the smaller teeth, suggests that the digestive system had become smaller. And the only way that their gut could become smaller, according to Professor Aiello, was with a high quality diet, e.g. eating high-energy foodstuffs, things that they could digest easily and could extract the nutrients from in a small length of intestinal tissue. This relationship, the gut becoming smaller and the brain becoming larger "seems magical to me" I wondered aloud, "that somehow, our bodies would know to do this…"

"It's not magic; it's evolution. And it's evolution because those individuals that got it right are the ones that reproduced, produced the offspring, and actually spread their genes into the next generation."

Certainly, this evolutionary pattern of body form changes and diet seems to have been the right formula for them at this period of time. Because it's during this time, right after our ancestors achieved this change in their body form and the inferred change in diet, that they began to migrate out of Africa. And the next place we pick them up again in the archaeological record is in the Far East, and then later on, in Europe.

The Next Big Change

Our brain and body sizes didn't really change much during the period 2 million to 1.6 million years ago. In fact, not much happened again for another million years. But then, at about a half million years before the present (BP), our journey to the becoming human story takes off again.

"About a half million years ago, things begin to change again and the brain begins to expand…. This is a period where we have ancestors called homo heidelburgensis appear. Now, we don't really know why this happens and it's one of the big mysteries in human evolution. But it's this type of ancestor that seems to be more successful in the more northern latitudes, like into Europe…and it's this type of ancestor, in general terms, we think are the antecedents, the predecessors, of the famous Neanderthal man."

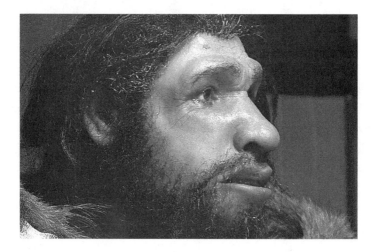

According to the *Natural History Museum* in London, the evidence suggests that the African *Homo heidelbergensis* could be the ancestor of both the Neanderthals and Modern Humans. *Homo heidelbergensis* is known to have lived in both Africa and Europe. They routinely butchered large animals and their fossil remains are often associated with hand axes.

Modern Humans First Appearance

What an anthropologist would term as "anatomically modern humans" would be people that had heads like ours that were very rounded, with small faces tucked under the brain case, with the long linear body form. These types of individuals first appear in Africa about 160,000 years ago; so in the entire course of evolutionary history it's quite recent.

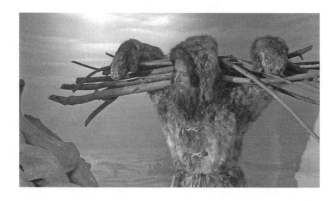

Big Brains = *Smarter than all the Rest*?

With those big brains that were part of our development, it begs the question, with those bigger brains, were we smarter? *"Yes, is the short answer,"* Professor Aiello said. The longer answer is that it's a very difficult thing for these scientists to know because current modern humans have a huge range of body sizes and a huge range of brain sizes. And, similarly, we would expect our early ancestors would have had similar range both in body and brain sizes.

Part of what I learned on my search for the solution to obesity and diet-related disease is that scientists, researchers and academics are very reluctant to take the position that they have the final word in any area of research or study. What appears to be ingrained in many of them is that they are in a constant state of discovery and of learning new things. Therefore, even when there appears to be a definitive answer, they always leave the door open, at least a little bit, insinuating that they haven't learned it all yet.

Professor Aiello was quick to point out that when we say big brains equal greater intelligence, that she was not saying that a person with a smaller brain than you have is stupider than you are, or vice versa.

> *"If we're looking at it across species, we assume that the increase in brain size, as we track it from our earliest ancestors all the way through to modern humans, actually tracks a change in cognitive ability. And of course one of the big things here is the evolution of language, because this is something that does separate us from our closest living relatives."*

An interesting question is, in addition to cognitive[17] ability (conscious mental activities like thinking, understanding, learning and remembering), could our development of a spoken language also have helped influence the increased brain size?

---

17   http://www.merriam-webster.com/dictionary/cognition

"There has to be a relationship. I mean, if I had to put my money on it I'd say that this increase in brain size at about a half million years ago is tracking the evolution of language. But there are other opinions, and there's really no hard evidence to test it right now."

Human Body Fat

Professor Aiello said that the foods modern humans ate was an ideal diet in good times, but these early ancestors also went through a number of bad times when it was difficult to find enough food. Much of that was directly related to the many dramatic climate changes that have occurred. Human body fat and our ability to store that fat is, in her view, a direct reaction to this fluctuation in food availability that our ancestors experienced throughout evolutionary history. For example, modern humans arrived in Europe during what is called an "interstitial", meaning "between two cold periods." The weather is unstable and irregular; sometimes it is quite cold and at other times temperate. In addition, modern humans arrived in Europe before the last glacial event, which peaks about 18,000 to 20,000 years ago, which is one of the coldest moments ever experienced by humans who lived in this area.

Obesity & Fat Babies

One thing we know is that humans have larger amounts of body fat than other primates. We also know that human females have larger amounts of body fat than their male counterparts. And human babies at birth have the largest percentage of body fat of all three. And why? Because body fat supports the growth and development of the brain, much of which happens in the first five years of life. And it is that ability to store body fat that helped us ascend the evolutionary ladder.

If you look at human obesity in this context, you see that our early ancestors went through cyclical periods of plenty and famine. They would store fat during good times for use during lean times. In addition to individual survival, the larger percentage of body fat in women is a very important mechanism. Females not only have to provide energy for themselves, but also for infants they might be gestating. And for early modern human females it was particularly important during lactation, which was a much longer period in prehistory than in current modern humans. And so, what was our fat? It was and still is genetic insurance. But what's happened today is that we no longer need that insurance. It just builds up and builds up and builds up, ultimately leading to obesity.

> *"There's sort of tantalizing things that we see in the archaeological record. In the Upper Paleolithic during the ice age in Europe you have these beautiful little Venus figurines...these are images of the female body, and they're all... we would term them 'obese.' And this was apparently an ideal form in the Upper Paleolithic.*
>
> *If you look at this in terms of insurance, those women with this type of body form would be those that would survive the difficult periods. And, you know, who knows? It gets into speculation... but at least they knew of overweight people."*

The Beginning of Our Decline

There are a number of stories about what constituted ideal human nutrition I remember from my childhood. The one that comes to mind immediately is that we, current modern humans, started out smaller and shorter way back in time, and because of the miracle of having better nutrition than we had in the past, we are now bigger, stronger and healthier than ever before. Turns out that this story isn't true. And there are a couple of reasons for this: 1) we have been told that "longevity" means we're healthier. This belief is predicated on more sophisticated medical interventions that extend life even in the face of disease and extremely poor health, and 2) culturally we tend to define "before" in terms of a few generations before our lifetime, not in millennial terms of our species evolution.

When it comes to being bigger, stronger and healthier in relation to our journey becoming human, what we know now is many of the earliest modern humans were very big, tall and robust individuals. And contrary to the persistent myth that they all had short lives, often with the implication that it's because they weren't healthy, skeletons of individuals who lived as long as our current average life spans have been found. As you'll see a bit later in chapter 7, the health and longevity problems they faced were due to very different reasons than ours, not poor nutrition.

> *"One of my old professors used to say this (the late Paleolithic) was the high period of human evolution and it's been downhill since then because they were eating a huge diversity of food stuffs...(For example) we go to the supermarket, and when we make a salad we think that we're eating a lot of different types of veggies and all, but in comparison to what our early ancestors were eating, this isn't true.... they had a huge diversity."*

Beginning 10,000 years ago we see our skeletons becoming less robust. The fossil evidence clearly shows a dramatic decrease in stature and skeletal strength during the last five to 10,000 years, beginning in the Middle East and slowly spreading around the globe. That major change happened with the development and gradual adoption of grain-based agriculture, which of course is a total change in the early modern human diet.

> *"Once you start agriculture, you seriously reduce the variety in your food and this also reduces the variety of nutrients you get. And what we think we're seeing when we see the real reduction in the skeletons, when we see evidence in the skeletons of nutritional deficiency, that what we're tracking is this reduction of variation in the diet."*

I mentioned to Professor Aiello that a number of the experts I had interviewed said similar things; that our species' decline in health started with the advent of agriculture and its displacement of critical animal proteins and fats.

> *"Of course... we aren't getting what we were built to need... and I think that's the bottom line of it."*

Our Species' Current Dilemma

In America today somewhere between three and four hundred thousand people a year are dying because of obesity and obesity related diseases[18]. And tragically, the obesity epidemic and diet related chronic disease is rapidly spreading to other modern countries that adopt our foods and way of life. A short list of diet related chronic diseases include: inflammatory and autoimmune diseases, diabetes, CAD (coronary artery disease), high blood pressure and some types of cancer.

For the most part, we have plenty of "foods" widely available in westernized countries, although most of the foods we find at the local supermarket are packaged and highly processed, refined convenience foods. I asked Professor Aiello if the crux of our current obesity problem is that important ability to store body fat for times of survival, and now, we've just got too much food easily available?

"Well, yes, basically. I mean we have too much, and we aren't active enough. I mean we aren't living the lifestyle that I believe we were evolved to live because if you look at evolutionary history we've got these seven million years it's taken us to get here. And the obesity epidemic has kicked in the last ten, twenty, thirty years, forty years; it's a very, very short time in evolutionary history. And in that same period of time we've had the increase in abundance...we've also, of course, had the spread of cars where, you know, everyone has at least one car now, and that's not helping us physically."

This is an important and fundamental evolutionary understanding about our species when considering the causes and solutions of obesity at this stage in our human story. Lack of daily movement and exercise coupled with the year-round and over abundant food supply in our modern world, is not in sync with our body's seven million year-old hardwiring.

---

18   "What is distressing or painful about a dilemma is having to make a choice one does not want to make." http://www.merriam-webster.com/dictionary/dilemma

"I'm just surprised we made it"

As we were nearing the end of our conversation I shifted gears a bit, as had become my habit with these scientific interviews, turning the questions from professional to personal. The way Professor Aiello answered them was so thoughtful I wanted you to have a chance to experience her responses as she expressed them to me. These last three questions are transcribed from our filmed interview.

CJ: "Asking you to step out of academia, the science, right now; just as a woman living in New York, just for yourself, how do you feel about all of this? The obesity epidemic? And do you think we can stop it?"

Professor Aiello: *"Can you stop anything humans do? I mean yes in an ideal world we can stop it, we can stop people smoking, we can change behavior. The question is, we can't do this for everyone or everyone won't want it done. And what's going to happen is… this is actually evolution in action. Well, shall we say if you weren't physiologically adapted to carrying around the extra weight, you aren't going to be successful in evolutionary terms, you aren't going to have as many kids, you aren't going to get as many genes into the next generation. So evolution is going to adjust.*

"But it's the artificial environment that we live in (that can change this outcome), because one of the main differences between ourselves and our early ancestors is we create our own environment around us as we go. So where our early ancestors used tools, and in this way were creating a small artificial environment around themselves, we have a huge artificial environment around us, and we have quite sophisticated medical knowledge.

"Now, if we can intervene and make these people invisible to evolution, then evolution isn't going to act in terms of prohibiting or restricting the reproduction of these individuals, causing them to die earlier."

CJ: "Where they are sorted out of the gene pool?"

Professor Aiello: *"It's possible that culture will not allow them to be sorted out of the gene pool, you know, with medical intervention.*

"But, I'm just surprised we made it... because when you look at the record there are so many periods in human evolution where we think that there were bottlenecks. Where it was... it was sort of very close whether we actually made it through a particular crisis... and, you know, then, we're on course again. And I'm sure many, many, many, small groups of early humans died out. But there were always other small groups that then came in to replace them.

If you model mortality and various assumptions of survivorship in early human evolution, it looks like they were fairly close to the edge in many, many, time periods."

CJ: "So, maybe they can give us hope. If we're really close to the edge again for a different reason, that we can figure our way out of it with those big brains."

Professor Aiello: *"We would hope so."*

Reporter's Notebook

Becoming Human:

1. Approximately 2-million years ago, our early ancestors began eating more animal-based foods, e.g. bone marrow, brains.
2. These foods provided the nutrients and long chain fatty acids for brain growth.
3. Anatomically modern humans first appeared about 160,000 years ago in Africa, quite recently in evolutionary history.
4. Ability to store body fat is a survival adaptation—insurance for lean times—particularly for females who might be eating for two (gestation and lactation periods).

Agricultures Effects:

1. Agriculture seriously reduced the variety in our food, reducing the variety of nutrients in our diet.
2. Our skeletons changed radically due to these nutritional deficiencies; e.g. we lost height, our bones less robust, smaller skulls, dental cares, etc.
3. We are at a disadvantage by not having the wide variety of food possibilities that our ancestors had.

The Bottom Line... We aren't getting what we were built to need—the right foods and sufficient physical movement.

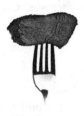

THINK EVOLUTION:
THE HARD EVIDENCE

Chapter 5

"We do not know how to eat properly. We feed ourselves, but we fail to give ourselves the proper nutrition. And after a while it becomes cumulative, and that's when we start developing degenerative diseases."
—**Gary J. Sawyer**, Physical Anthropologist,
American Museum of Natural History

A s I was wrapping up the interview with Professor Aiello, she said: *"You know who you should go talk to is,"* then she mentioned the scientists at the American Museum of Natural History's Division of Anthropology there in New York. Behind the scenes, the museum has a lab where they create forensic reconstructions of our ancestors based on fossils that have been recovered from various dig sites worldwide. She felt this would be of particular interest to me because the reconstructions are built based on what the forensic reconstruction team knows about the foods these ancestors were eating. And because they know this, they are able to better approximate the size of the body, the shape and details of the musculature and skin in order to produce more accurate recreations.

As it turned out, the *American Museum of Natural History* was ready to open its new Spitzer Hall of Human Origins. If I could get permission from the museum, it would be a great location to shoot some footage of the artifacts, fossils and reconstructions of the ancestors Professor Aiello and I had just discussed, including the museum's many dioramas depicting scenes from our ancestral past. More importantly, it would be a rare opportunity to get further insight into the *becoming human* story that could have beneficial applications for you and me to significantly improve our health and well-being.

After several emails and phone calls, I was gratified to hear back from the Museum press-relations office approving my filming in the new exhibit. They had also arranged for me to interview Gary J. Sawyer, a physical anthropologist in the museum's Division of Anthropology.

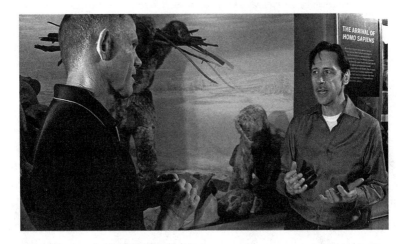

Mr. Sawyer had been involved in the development of numerous exhibits at the museum, specializing in the forensic reconstruction of our extinct relatives, all of which are based on the most up-to-date evidence of where— and how—our ancestors lived. His distinguished career includes leading the team that created the first-ever complete reconstruction of a Neanderthal skeleton.

He and I decided to start the interview at the point where our early ancestor, Homo erectus (meaning upright man), was starting to incorporate more animal foods into their diet, about two million years ago. As we walked over to one of the new dioramas, he told me, *"We're now going to take a big leap in time into what we call the early Paleolithic."* Stopping a few inches from a large glass wall he continued, *"We're now two million years into the past... What I'd like to point out is the environment where these people lived. All open grassland, what we call savanna. There are trees in the background, but it's very open, very dangerous territory for them."*

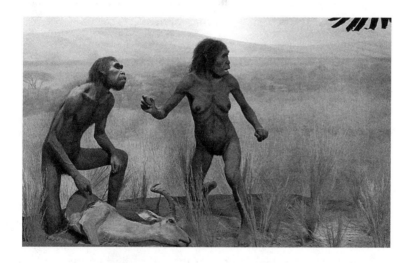

It was fascinating to see this often used scientific description of the savanna come to life in 3D, particularly from a team known for creating compellingly accurate representations. Mr. Sawyer explained some of the details of their lifestyle, and also some of the physical similarities to modern humans that anthropologists have pieced together. Walking, they had a stride that was more like ours than those of earlier ancestors, and they ran like us as well. And brainpower? Were these individuals as intelligent as you and me? "No, they weren't" he said. "But they probably had instincts that you and I have long since lost."

One of the most interesting things about this moment in our history is that these ancient people, as primitive as they were, were already making sophisticated tools. We know they were primarily scavengers; hunting behaviors had yet to be developed. To dramatize this for visitors to the exhibit, Mr. Sawyer and his team created a snapshot of what the Homo erectus couples daily life was like on the savanna.

In the diorama pictured above, you can see a man holding a primitive flint tool fashioned for cutting. He is distracted from cutting into the side of a freshly killed antelope by attacking predators, while at the same time his female companion tries to scare off the attack by these opportunists. Life was not easy in the savanna for our ancestors. Nevertheless, that environment provided exactly the nutritional elements they needed to keep our *becoming human* story moving forward.

> *"These people were now becoming more and more meat eaters, and we feel that this had a great deal to do with expansion of the brain. Our bodies evolved (into) the way they are now quickly. Our brain… took a while to catch up. However with a high protein diet, that's what they had, that was the secret for encephillating*[19] *(growing) our brain… and for the greater intelligence that we have today."*

Mr. Sawyer pointed out that the secret behind their brain growth was two-fold; the leap that they made from earlier ancestors' vegetarianism to an animal sourced, higher protein diet with the important addition of essential fats and cholesterol. They acquired that fat and cholesterol by cracking open the skulls of these animals to get to the brain tissue (which is high in cholesterol) and by breaking open the long bones to get to the marrow. His point was that, already, two million years ago, early fossil humans were consuming meat and animal fats, and that momentous

---

19   In Zoology: (NOUN) An evolutionary increase in the complexity or relative size of the brain, involving a shift of function from non-cortical parts of the brain to the cortex. Source: http://www.oxforddictionaries.com/us/definition/american_english/encephalization

upgrade in nutrition made a big difference in our evolution, and how our brains developed.

"We believe it made all the difference in our evolution. If we had stayed as vegetarians, in all probability, I wouldn't be speaking to you on this particular high level of intellect."

The Last Human

During a short break in between shots, I took a look around the Hall of Human Origins to see what the Anthropology division had gathered to illustrate and explain human evolution, the complete *becoming human* story. Our story can be seen in a rather complex tree representing our history. One of the most interesting displays showed a selection of the actual fossil evidence retracing the last two million years until it reached our time, present day modern humans, "Homo sapiens." [20] I didn't realize that we now know of 22 distinct species in our history, many of them coexisting in the world at the same time, and they are all now extinct. Present day modern humans are the only ones that survived.

"In my opinion it was a grand experiment by nature and natural selection, with you and me the final product. It was a matter of competition; it was a matter of natural selection; it was a matter of the environment. It was many factors that went into making us unique, different from all the others."

Evolution: *The Hard Evidence*

I asked Mr. Sawyer what was the most compelling artifact he has come across in his study of evolution and anthropology? A few minutes later he returned with a small black box and placed it on a display table in front of us. As he opened the box, he said, *"What I'd like to do now is show you something that we call 'the hard evidence of human evolution'."* I watched him lift an ancient skull out of that box, and for just for an instant it looked to

---

20   The name comes from the Greek "Homo," meaning "same," and Latin "sapiens," meaning "to know."

me like it might be a prop from a recent major Hollywood movie. It was fascinating, and over the next few moments it became even more so. This ancient skull was here at the Museum and it wasn't a Hollywood prop, it was a *real* (you can see it below).

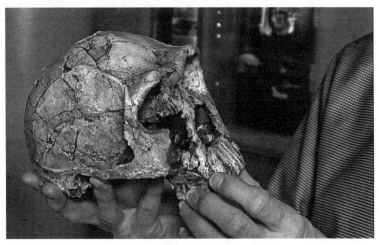

Continuing, he said,

> *"This is a fossilized skull[21], approximately two million years old, in excellent condition. To find a specimen like this so perfectly preserved... is telling us a great deal. These ancient humans have left behind a record in the crust of the earth and they're actually now beginning to speak to us. It's identifiable, so to speak, as a human skull. It's definitely part human, part primitive. We do see an expansion in the brain case, but nothing compared to the expansion in our brain case."*

As you can see in the picture from the film,[22] the skull has very large brow ridges, which you and I have lost because our cranium has expanded

---

21 Found in Kenya.

22 The diorama project team uses real fossil evidence like this skull to construct these lifelike re-creations in the exhibit. In fact, compare this ancient skull with the head of the male Homo erectus in the diorama and you can easily see how the project team has utilized it as a model for his head.

considerably. Another easily noticeable evolutionary change is that our forehead has gone from low and sloped, to straight up and down.

> *"It's just fantastic that nature has left behind the evidence, what we call 'the hard evidence', proving conclusively that at least two million years ago there was a creature that was neither fully human, neither fully modern, but certainly on the road to becoming us. We have indeed evolved as humans."*

Modern Humans

Mr. Sawyer then walked me over to another of the new dioramas, this one featuring anatomically modern humans. They were still very primitive at this time, but otherwise just like you and me. As you can see below, these modern humans are living in a cold tundra environment and have constructed a home that is made of mammoth bones (inspired by an actual site).

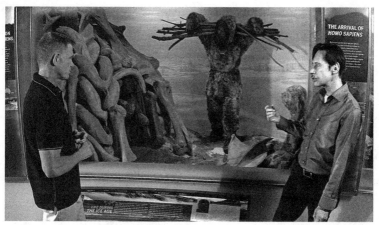

This couple is living roughly 30 to 40 thousand years before the present (BP). They are still making their tools out of stone and bone; no metal exists. Yet, modern humans are advancing considerably, innovating clothes sewn with bone needles to protect themselves from the harsh environment, and a primitive form of refrigeration taking advantage of the frozen ground to bury meat for future use. This is just before the beginning of agriculture. Just before a big change in human evolution.

> *"These are what we call anatomically modern humans just like you and me, identical in all respects; same form of intelligence, everything. However, they're still living in the Paleolithic, which means that their diet so to speak is lean meat, fish, any form of vegetation they could get, fruits, berries, nuts. Everything is coming from a world that was pristine as opposed to a world today that is highly polluted."*

Mr. Sawyer feels if modern humans had stayed in this pristine state, it's very unlikely we would have the diseases we're seeing today. Their diet was simple: "lean" meat, fats; internal organs, marrow, brains and fish. And some seasonal plant foods like fruit, nuts and berries. This kind of diet, the foods they ate during the pre-agricultural age, was nutritionally superior. After that, our species starts to decline.

My last question brought us back to what is a central concept in the *becoming human* story, and of my search for the perfect human diet. "The foods that were available to them in nature is what helped move evolution forward, right?"

> *"I believe so, definitely. It was a struggle. It was survival of the fittest. And today we are it. We are the end product of that long survival."*

Reporter's Notebook

Homo erectus (early ancestor):

1. Approx. 2 million years ago, living in African savanna.
2. Stood upright. Similar stride and run.
3. Primarily scavengers.
4. Already making sophisticated tools.
5. Began eating more animal-based foods, e.g. bone marrow, brains.
6. Animal foods responsible for brain growth.

Anatomically Modern Humans:

1. On display, recent moderns. 30-40 k years ago.
2. Stone and bone tools. No metal yet.
3. Created clothes sewn with bone needles.
4. Diet muscle meat ("lean"), fats; organs, marrow, brains, fish. Seasonal plant foods, e.g., fruit, nuts and berries.
5. This diet was nutritionally superior. Pristine world, unpolluted.
6. Diet changed with agriculture, we started to decline.

Evolution's Scientific Proof:

1. Rare fossilized skull, approximately 2,000,000 years old.
2. Part human, part primitive.

The Bottom Line... *Present day modern humans are the only survivors of 22 versions. Survival of the fittest.*

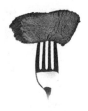

THINK TREASURE:
EXACTLY LIKE US

Chapter 6

"Well, fortunately they were healthy... because we would not be here, if they were not healthy."
> —**Professor Marie Soressi**, Max Planck
> Institute of Evolutionary Anthropology

In early 2006, I repeatedly heard the same words after the completion of every interview: "You know who you should talk to is ..." followed by the name of a scientist or researcher I'd never heard of, but who possessed a crucial expertise that might help me in my search. This is also the occasion where I first heard there was new technology that can tell us *exactly* what humans ate in the past— no more theories, just scientific facts. As a journalist-filmmaker, I was excited and intrigued to learn about this recent scientific innovation that could reveal archeological details that were previously unknowable.

Well, we've all heard the "be careful what you ask for" stories, and this unexpected opportunity turned out to be located at the *Max Planck Institute for Evolutionary Anthropology*, in Leipzig, Germany. I had one brief moment of pause upon hearing this, as I was still a college student getting by on small school loans and trying to finance this treasure hunt out of my own pocket. Nevertheless, I called up Professor Mike Richards, director of the Anthropological Sciences Department at the Institute, to see if he would be willing to be interviewed for the film. Not only was he willing, but he suggested I visit one of his department's active digs that summer in the south of France before coming to see him. Starting there would enable me to interview additional experts from their team, and *"follow the bones back to the lab"* in Leipzig where they are analyzed— a unique opportunity to film the human nutrition discovery process from start to finish. And of course, you never know what unexpected things you will discover if you are open to follow the story where it leads you. Little did I know how important this trip would be.

A few months later I found myself a short distance north of Bordeaux, France, standing in the middle of a fascinating archaeological dig site, described as *"the site of Jonzac,"* by Paleolithic archaeologist Professor Shannon McPherron, when he introduced me to the site.

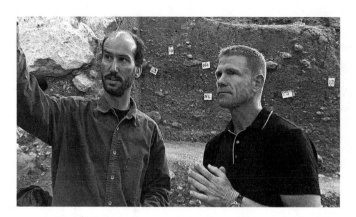

He continued my introduction by saying:

> *"They came here… they were butchering these animals… they were leaving behind the bones and the stone tools. We want to know a little bit more about that. Were they cutting off the meaty parts and taking those with them? Do you find evidence of those parts still here? What exactly was the process that lead to the creation of this thick deposit of bones?"*

The Jonzac site (also called Chez Pineau[23]) is a Middle Paleolithic[24] and early Upper Paleolithic[25] site that was discovered accidentally just over 100 years ago when local people cut a road through a hillside to access limestone, which they then quarried for building material. The exposed walls of earth on either side of the road cut revealed a number of very rich layers of artifacts and bones. But interestingly enough, they didn't report it to officials. The discovery didn't make it into any publications. And the site went unnoticed again for about 100 years. Then in the 1990s, a French geologist working in the region came to the site, noticed the stone tools and the bones in the layers, and brought it to the attention of a local archeologist who realized the importance of the find. Now, the Max Planck team was back working the site for the third (and last) time to explore this rich archaeological find.

In The Dig: *Success Leaves Clues*
In addition to a large bed of animal bones the team was excavating, one of the most interesting things about the site is the many layers on both

23 The Jonzac site is located on the property of Chez Pineau, a former cognac distillery and sits in the shadow of the Château de la Dîmerie estate and winery.

24 The Middle Paleolithic, or Middle *Stone Age* (ca 200,000 to 45,000 years ago or so), is the period during which Archaic humans including Neanderthals appeared and flourished all over the world. Soruce: http://archaeology.about.com/od/mterms/qt/middle_paleolit.htm

25 The Upper Paleolithic, or *Late Stone Age*, is the third and last subdivision of the Paleolithic (Old Stone Age). It dates to between 50,000 and 10,000 years ago, roughly coinciding with the appearance of behavioral modernity and before the advent of agriculture. Source: http://en.wikipedia.org/wiki/Upper_Paleolithic

sides of the roadbed, much of which is straight up and down like the walls of a room. The layers encompass three distinct time periods, starting at the floor of the dig and progressing upwards to the most recent time at the top of the wall: 1) the long period when Neanderthals inhabited the area, 2) the short time when modern humans entered the picture; artifacts from both groups share some of the limestone layers, and 3) the last and most recent layer representing only modern humans (The Neanderthals had disappeared).

The team looks for artifacts that help reconstruct the diets of Neanderthals and modern humans. In order to reconstruct that diet, they retrieve and study the bones and stone tools left behind in the layers by both groups. Professor McPherron explained that the primitive stone tools they were finding, such as "scrapers" and hand-axes, were used for butchering food animals brought back from hunting.

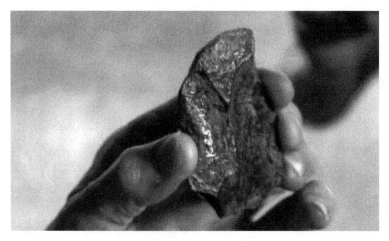

Stone Scraper Tool

He said, "When you see this (stone) technology, you can spot it. It has certain characteristics that we can easily identify. And in a lot of sites in this region it's associated with these kinds of bone bed deposits."

Of course I was very interested in anything they found in the site that would tell us about the diet of the modern humans who lived there. I wanted to know things like what kinds of animals they hunted, and if all the bones I could see the team recovering were animal bones (there were lots of them).

> *"Yep, all animal bones, and mostly reindeer. There are some horse… and there are some bison as well. But it's mostly reindeer, meaning that they were probably in a cold period at this point in time. Then we get a series of layers that are not as rich, but tend to have the same kinds of bones and the same kinds of stone tools."*

One thing the researchers have lots of evidence for is marrow extraction: breaking the bones open to get the marrow out. Learning this, I asked the professor if there was there anything else the team was recovering, in addition to that evidence, which could explain very specifically what foods they ate?

> *"The evidence, for the most part, is going to come from the bones because that's what's preserved. We can talk later about isotopic studies[26] that…give you a different line of evidence in the diet. But here, what we're looking at are mostly large mammals. As I said, reindeer, and then there's some evidence of a shift towards the top of our sequence (the period of modern humans replacing Neanderthals)… towards some horse and some bison."*

It's interesting to note what animals that could have been food sources in these periods, but are missing from the site. Particularly since there is a common assumption that modern humans, as opportunists, would eat anything they could get their hands on wherever they were located. But in actuality, Neanderthals and modern humans both appear to have had clear preferences for certain food sources over others when they could get them, just like we do in our time. Mostly, they preferred medium-sized to large mammals. Missing, were small mammals such as rabbit, and small carnivores like fox. Birds, especially, were very rare and you don't find a lot of fish in their diets either. For example, I was told in a follow-up call

---

26   Presented in Chapter 8.

with the Department of Human Evolution in 2014 that recent research[27] revealed that early modern humans living around the Mediterranean Sea did *not* exploit seafood. Contrary to popular belief, marine resources were not important foods in their diet at that time. "The source of the dietary protein consumed mainly originated from the meat of medium to large terrestrial herbivores," said Marcello Mannino, an archaeologist at the *Max Planck Institute for Evolutionary Anthropology.*

I asked Professor McPherron if there is anything especially unique about the food remains at the Jonzac dig site, he replied saying, "Not really." He said that just 30 minutes to the East was another dig site similar to Jonzac, and instead of reindeer as the apparent food of choice it was bison and horse. But again, at that dig site the dietary preference was for large mammals. That fact, and the fact that the artifacts of food animals remained the same in all layers of the Jonzac dig site, supported what I'd been learning about our species actively hunting animal foods. Even after the disappearance of the Neanderthal. But even more interesting was what Professor McPherron said as our discussion continued.

Professor McPherron: *"You don't find Neanderthals after that layer… the moderns came in."*

CJ: "So modern humans, more like us?"

Professor McPherron: *"Yes, exactly like us."*

CJ: *"Exactly* like us?"

Professor McPherron: *"Yes…at least in terms of what we can say about their biology, exactly like us. And when we look at the archaeology, they had a range of cultural behavior that we would say is modern. They were modern humans. They had a brain that was organized, as far as we can tell, like ours.*

---

27   Origin and Diet of the Prehistoric Hunter-Gatherers on the Mediterranean Island of Favignana (Ègadi Islands, Sicily) Marcello A. Mannino et al Published: November 28, 2012 http://www.plosone.org/article/info:doi/10.1371/journal.pone.0049802

They did different things of course, but they had that potential to do the same range of the kinds of things that we do today."

Agriculture

Before we wrapped up the shoot, I asked the professor one last question: Was there was any evidence of agriculture at this site?

He noted that the top layer of the excavation dated back to about 10,000 years ago, which coincided with early humans adopting agriculture. But grain and plant agriculture started in the Near East and took many years [28] to work its way into Western Europe. The people in this part of the world were still hunter-gatherers whose main diet was medium to large game animals.

The Elephant in the Room: *Were they Healthy?*

I also had a chance to talk with another senior member of the team— Professor Marie Soressi.

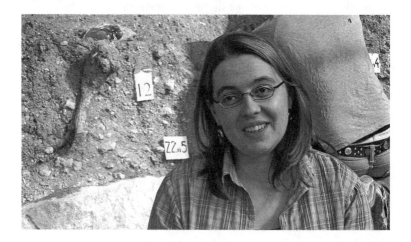

Currently, Professor Soressi is a researcher at the French National Institute for Preventive Archaeology, where she is responsible for Paleolithic excavations in the center of France. Her main interests include research

---

28 Upwards of 5,000 years.

into what behaviors contributed to the success of anatomically modern humans in Europe.

Of course, one of the big questions brought up repeatedly by the media in our time is whether or not we should use early modern humans and their diet as a guideline for our own health. Her answer was as straightforward as one could get, and charming through her French accent.

CJ: "Professor Soressi, would you say, based on the archaeological evidence that they (modern humans) were healthy compared to humans today?"

Professor Soressi: *"Well, fortunately they were healthy… because we would not be here, if they were not healthy."*

Reporter's Notebook

Jonzac Dig site:

1. First Neanderthals, replaced by modern humans.
2. Neanderthals made stone tools and were butchering animals on the site.
3. Mostly reindeer, suggesting they were in a cold period.
4. Neanderthal and modern humans were good hunters by this point.
5. Lots of evidence for marrow extraction.
6. Modern humans only in recent, upper layers (No Neanderthals).

Animals Found:

1. Other large animals butchered here, horse and bison.

Animals Missing:

1. Small mammals, rabbit, birds (very rare), not a lot of fish.
2. No evidence of agriculture at this site. Much later. 25k yrs. or so towards the present.

The Bottom Line... *The modern humans who came to Europe were "exactly like us" – they were healthy and they're eating primarily medium-large sized mammals.*

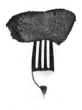

THINK SURVIVOR:
OUR PLACE IN NATURE

Chapter 7

"Well, I'm sure that they had a lot of troubles with their health, but very different kinds of problems than what we have now."
—**Jean-Jacques Hublin**, Director,
Department of Human Evolution, Max Planck Institute

A ll of the fossils and artifacts[29] excavated at the site of Jonzac are taken a few miles away to a temporary field lab where team members identify, bag, label and log everything that was recovered prior to the journey back to the Department of Human Evolution's laboratories in Leipzig, Germany. The department itself is an international team, bringing together a wide variety of people who are interested in different aspects of human history during this timeframe. Those interests include the evolution of human biology, human behavior and human culture.

29　In archaeology, an object formed by humans, e.g. stone tools.

I went to the Jonzac field lab to meet with the head of the department, Professor Jean-Jacques Hublin. I wanted to get his perspective about early modern human diet and lifestyle, our place in nature, and how the knowledge gleaned from this research might help us solve the significant health problems facing our species in our modern world.

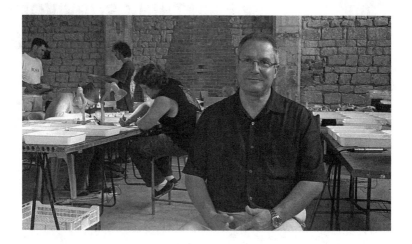

Initially, Professor Hublin's research focused on the origin and evolution of Neanderthals. That early research has now been expanded and includes the evolutionary processes that led to the emergence of modern humans in Africa, and the activities of their descendants, the anatomically modern humans in Europe. To facilitate the department's research, he developed the use of medical and virtual imaging to study our lineage, particularly in relation to our brain and cognitive abilities.

Jonzac is not the first dig site led by Professor Hublin, over the course of his career the professor has participated in over 15 archaeological excavations. With his having a uniquely broad professional background, I was curious to hear not only his assessment on what I had heard from other experts,[30] but what new elements he might bring forward that could help answer the most important questions about human

---

30 None of them had any prior knowledge of what had been said by the others.

diet and health. I started by asking him what the team was doing at Jonzac.

"Well, we are looking at a very peculiar moment in the evolution of humans in Europe. The moment when archaic forms of humans, the Neanderthals, went extinct and were replaced by modern humans, moderns looking just like us."

During the time when Neanderthals and the first modern humans lived in Western Europe, and when they lived at Jonzac, they were surrounded by many different kinds of animals due to the spectacular climate changes. During warmer episodes, prior to and including the arrival of modern humans in Europe, we see hunting for animals which are found in heavily forested, temperate environments, such as bison, aurochs[31] and horses (We find all these animals in the Jonzac site). In much colder periods after modern humans arrived, it was an environment similar to what we have today in Scandinavia or Siberia, and they hunted animals like reindeer, mammoth and woolly rhinoceros.

"Most of what we find in this kind of site is related to the diet, actually, because, primarily what we find is bone remains of the animals that have been killed by humans, their hunters. We also find all the artifacts that have been used to kill them, and to butcher them afterwards.

"So, there is primary evidence, which is this: one, we have an idea of what kind of animals they were interested in, and two, Neanderthals, like modern humans, were hunters of large mammals. They were, mostly, interested in large mammals. What's different with modern humans (is), they broadened their spectrum, a little bit, being interested in other kinds of food."

---

31 A large wild Eurasian ox that was the ancestor of domestic cattle. It was probably exterminated in Britain in the Bronze Age, and the last one was killed in Poland in 1627. Source: Apple Mac Dictionary 2014.

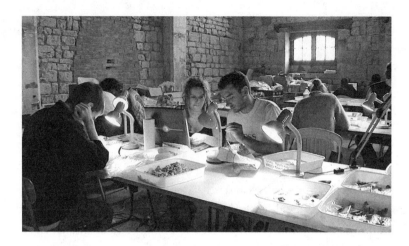

We don't know much about plant foods from direct evidence recovered from the dig sites, but archaeologists suspect that modern humans were also eating things like berries when they were available. At some sites there is direct evidence they gathered a variety of small vertebrates such as birds and fish, but the lion's share remains large land mammals.

Our Health

It's no secret that in our lifetime a heavily promoted message has declared that meat and animal fats are inherently unhealthy. Of course once we have all of the known science available to consider, including our new knowledge of what was previously unknowable, the question must be asked: If modern humans evolved as hunter-gatherers, becoming bigger, stronger and smarter, while eating primarily animal foods, were we healthy? Were we healthier then, than we are now?

One of the arguments against using human evolutionary nutrition as a model for regaining our health today is *"they didn't live very long"*, often expressed in the media[32] with an assumption that what our ancestors ate

---

32 E.g. Recently Good Morning America's senior medical expert Dr. Richard Besser said, "The idea that the cavemen got it right -- if you look back, cavemen didn't live past their 30s. Just as the big picture, not the ones that I would pick as role models." http://abcnews.go.com/GMA/video/paleo-diet-gains-attention-summer-dieters-24259444

was the biggest contributor to those alleged shorter lives. Professor Hublin had a very simple way of explaining this common misunderstanding about their diet and health.

"Well, I'm sure that they had a lot of troubles with their health, but (they had) very different kinds of problems than what we have now. We live in a society which is very safe; we don't have many accidents. Although we have violence, it's limited. And so, we're mainly preoccupied with all the health problems related to our diet and our way of life.

"I think, for the Neanderthals, or for the first modern humans in our region, they were mostly preoccupied with finding food. And the kind of problems they had in their daily lives with their health, was basically related to all the kinds of accidents they could have looking for food and hunting animals."

My follow-up question addressed obesity. Were they overweight? Was there obesity?

"What we can say, just looking at their skeletons, is that they were very tall, very strong, and very healthy people, in general. It's very unlikely that they had a lot of obesity. In their lives, they had to cope with a periodical shortage in the food supply. And it's very likely that many of our adaptations are related to this need to store fat during a period when we have a lot of food, and to be able to use this fat in shortage periods."

Body fat and women, a controversial subject of discussion in our modern times, but with the first modern humans in Europe, there have been a few small figurines found in the archeological record that suggest they might have felt differently about women and body fat. The professor noted that these small female statues indicate our ancestors seem appreciative of women who were plump, but not obese by contemporary standards.

"Maybe the idea they had about being obese was not the idea that we have today, which is considered a very problematic feature. Maybe in a society of hunter-gatherers, having to survive in a difficult time and environment, a woman with a lot of fat was something highly desirable."

The ability to store and use fat for energy was an important survival mechanism for both sexes. Females, especially, needed to be able to store enough extra fat to give birth to healthy babies during lean times, ensuring the survival of the species.

What was good for our species at that time, seems to be backfiring on us now with the growing epidemic of obesity and diet related chronic disease in westernized societies. And it's not getting any better because we're totally confused about how to eat in a way that will correct our downward spiral.

Clearly the evolutionary model says being able to store fat is crucial in case you face some period where you're not able to find food. The problem today is, of course, we can just sit in front of our TV or computer and store fat all year long. And most of the people living in developed societies don't face any kind of cyclical food shortage. Currently one of the big questions and public conflicts is that for more than 30 years we've been told that fats, especially animal fats, are bad for our health, and that grains are remarkably good for us (along with products made from grains, like cereals and bread). But recent ongoing nutritional research says loudly, NO; we got it wrong. There are some BIG problems with most of the foods we've been eating, especially since the agricultural revolution and the advent of modern processed foods, sugars and seed oils.

If that's true, from an evolutionary human nutrition perspective, where did we go wrong? Is there actually something wrong with most of the food we're eating?[33]

---

33   More than 70%. Source: *The Perfect Human Diet* documentary interview with Professor L. Cordain, Colorado State University.

For a long time, modern humans survived and thrived on a different type of food than what we have today. For several hundred thousand years, our ancestors had been primarily oriented to hunt animals, consuming their meat and their fat. Archaeologists believe they would also have had some small seasonal amounts of plant food, particularly in the warmer periods.

A very significant change started to occur to humans about 10,000 years ago when modern humans in the Mid East started to domesticate cereals, food animals, and develop farming. It was a great departure from their normal way of life. In fact we now know, those changes were a major revolution in human evolution—and in our shared human story.

The upside was that developing grain agriculture and domesticating animals allowed modern humans to have more security. They had more direct control over their food sources, and in particular, they could also store grains for consumption between growing seasons. But it also had a downside. While it provided increased security, it degraded the quality and variety of the foods available to them. One example of direct evidence for this is a reduction in our species body size between hunter-gatherers living 20,000 years ago, and farmers living 6,000 years ago. This change in body size shows up clearly in recovered fossils as a nutritional deficiency. The farmers became shorter, and, they acquired new health problems directly resulting from this fundamental change in their diet.

"We see a spectacular reduction in the body size between the last hunter-gatherers and the first farmers. People become shorter and they have all sorts of health problems that they did not have before. An explosion of cavities in the teeth, for example, (and) the frequency of cavities. And in general, the health status of this population does not seem so great.

"But this security allowed a very dramatic demographic development. In other words, hunter-gatherers were not numerous. (They were) a very limited population in the landscape, exploiting the fauna (the animals in a particular region)... and becoming farmers, they could become much more numerous... have villages...

some kind of security and a different mode of social organization. In the meantime, they have lost something, somehow.

From the farmers we have suffered some mis-adaptation[34] *related to the fact...that we're really not meant to eat so much cereal and sugar and things like that."*

Technology and Biology: *Strange Bedfellows*

Modern humans were immigrants, most likely coming from Africa. They invaded this region and out-competed the Neanderthals, eventually replacing them. This is a very significant moment in western Eurasia, because it's not just a biological revolution when one kind of human replaced another. It appears to be a major change in the social organization and adaptation of the technologies used by humans in their environment.

Humans are very special animals viewed through an evolutionary lens because in the beginning of our evolution, like other mammals, we were coping with environmental changes, mostly by the way of biological adaptation. We see many physical changes in our remote ancestors. About 2.5 million years ago, humans started to develop a lithic technology (stone technology). But not just stone technology, other technologies were very likely. As the professor said to me, *"What we see in the course of human evolution is that there is an increasing role of the technological, technical adaptation, and the decreasing importance of biological adaptation."*

That part of our human story, the technological advancements that made us able to live beyond the Arctic Circle for example, is nothing related to our biology. It is almost entirely because humans can build igloos and anoraks[35] and kayaks, which then allowed us to dwell on frozen lands. In the course of human evolution, we see a gradual change with more and more technical adaptations. And now we see this technological

---

34 The ability of a species to survive in a particular ecological niche, especially because of alterations of form or behavior brought about through natural selection. Biology http://dictionary.reference.com/browse/misadaptation

35 A waterproof jacket of a kind originally used in Polar Regions (typically with a hood). Source: Apple Dictionary 2014.

adaptation changing at such a speed that in the course of a single human life, we see spectacular changes. Unfortunately, these changes are not always to our benefit.

"Somehow, we have kept a body, which is the body of our ancestors 20,000 years ago that was hunting bison or reindeer. Who were roaming into the forests and the prairies....and our bodies are (now) a little bit out-run by this technological change."

Survival of the Fittest

Over the course of the 2.5 million years of history that we call the Paleolithic, there is a fact that isn't well known or understood by the general public. There was not just one single kind of human, but 22 distinct species of humans—of which we are the only one remaining.

As the professor clarified for me, *"I mean species as different as, let's say, chimpanzees and bonobos are different today"*—clearly identifiable differences.

This clarification prompted my last question to Professor Hublin. "Being the descendants of these early modern humans, the one that survived, are there things that we can learn from them? Things that could help us be healthier?"

"I think, in general, that it's very important to understand the past. As Cicero used to say 'Not to know what happened before you were born is to be a child forever' And I think it's true for prehistory, as well. We need to know something about our past evolution. To understand what our place in nature is, and what our fundamental adaptations are. I think that it's important to place all the questions about environment, the questions of demography and the questions about health, in general, in this broader context."

The modern humans that emerged about 150,000 - 200,000 years ago not only ended up populating the world, they (and now we) are the only surviving branch of a very complex tree. It's hard to ignore what seems self-evident. They must have been doing *something* right.

Reporter's Notebook

Big picture Jonzac:

1. Neanderthals looked like tall, strong, healthy people.
2. Like Neanderthals, modern humans were hunters of large animals.
3. Humans eventually broadened their spectrum a little, adding other foods, e.g., sm. vertebrates; fish, birds, berries.

Health:

1. Neanderthals different problems with health than we have.
2. In our time, we have health challenges related to our diet and way of life
3. Neanderthals preoccupied with finding food. Health problems related to accidents looking for and hunting food.
4. Modern humans able to store fat during abundant times to use in occasional shortages.
5. Now, Western society has an unlimited food supply. People can sit around and store fat continuously.

Agriculture's downside:

1. Farmers became shorter. Skeletons less robust.
2. General health declined.
3. Many health problems earlier humans did not have, e.g. explosion of cavities.

The Bottom Line... *There was not just one kind of human, but 22 distinct species of humans – of which we are the only one remaining. We are adapted to a different type of food. Our ancestors primarily oriented to hunt animals and consume their meat and fat.*

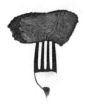

THINK WOW:
THE UNKNOWABLE BECOMES KNOWABLE

Chapter 8

"It's what evolutionary pressures pushed us towards, and we were successful in that kind of diet...It's got to be the best diet for humans."
—**Professor Mike Richards**, Max Planck Institute, Leipzig, Germany

I n 2003 I attended a scientific symposium at the *University of Arkansas* on the *"Evolution of the Human Diet; The Known, the Unknown, and the Unknowable"* that opened my eyes in a completely new way. I was surprised to hear the field of anthropology was just entering a period of exploding scientific understanding. For the first time, new technologies were shedding light on anthropological facts, including facts about the human diet, which were previously unknowable. It was an exciting and enlightening three days that left me wanting to know even more.

Three years after the symposium, I was in Leipzig, Germany, to interview Professor Mike Richards who I'd heard was not only an expert in the field, but using one of the most interesting scientific advancements realized to date—a method of analysis that uses biochemistry to look deep into the composition of the bones left behind by our ancestors. By analyzing our ancestors' bones with this new technology, scientists can tell us *exactly* what modern humans from locations all over the world ate on a regular basis. They can also tell us the diets of the animals and Neanderthals who lived in these sites, and even tell us exactly what modern humans were eating when our species' health began to decline. This new scientific ability, of course, is now an essential source of information to determine our species' past diet, at the time when we were much stronger and much healthier. Information that could help solve the major health problems we face today.

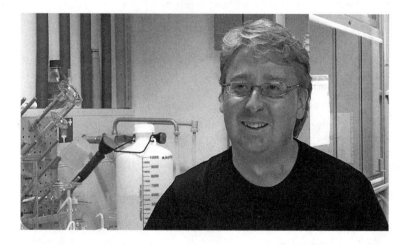

Mike Richards is a professor in the Department of Human Evolution at the *Max Planck Institute of Evolutionary Anthropology* where he runs the archaeological science group. His group specializes in applying hard science techniques to anthropological and archaeological questions. Professor Richards primary research interests are: reconstructing past diets, contrasting the diets of Neanderthals and modern humans in Europe, and the shift in diet associated with the adoption of agriculture.

"My main specialty is diet. I study bone chemistry as a way of getting at what the diets of people and animals were in the past. And one of the main things we're looking at is the evolution of diets, through time, by trying to get this information from these bones themselves, and by doing scientific analysis of the composition of these bones."

The fossils recovered from a dig site are called "the direct archeological evidence," and before this new technology's existence, archaeologists could only guess at what different foods modern humans might have eaten. Now that we can look directly at the proteins within the bones, it's finally possible to substantiate the actual food sources in the modern human diet before and after the adoption of agriculture.

"What it shows is what people hypothesized: it's a trait of our species that it's animal products which led to our increased brain size and all sort of other things which set us apart from other primates. And the problem has been that the evidence for this is circumstantial. You find tools that are being used to cut up animals. You find butchered animal bones. But there is no way to really tell what proportion of the diet that represented. And plant foods just don't survive, so they're invisible. So we have to use this kind of study, looking directly at the fossils themselves, the bone chemistry, to really prove what proportion of their diets was coming from animal protein versus plant protein."

How it's Done

The process begins by taking a sample, usually from a museum or from a dig site in the field. When the sample gets back to the lab, the outside layer is cleaned off, eliminating any contaminants from the soil. The bone is next placed into a hydrochloric acid solution. This dissolves away most of the bone, which is mineral, until what remains is the protein. The next few stages further filter and process the protein until only the collagen remains. Next, the scientists place the freeze-dried collagen into a mass spectrometer[36] and check for two things: one, the amount of carbon and nitrogen present in the sample to ensure that it's really collagen, and two, the isotopic ratio signature which identifies the food sources consumed. It is this ratio that allows for a comparison between herbivores and carnivores, and then how modern humans and Neanderthals fit into that comparison chart.

To further illustrate, the ratios from reindeer—a known herbivore—and the ratios from wolves - a known carnivore - possess dramatically different signatures and fall at the extreme ends of the chart. The isotopic ratio signatures of modern humans and Neanderthals who lived in that same area at the same time can then be placed on the comparison chart against the two known extremes - clearly identifying their diet.

"We then take those isotopic ratios and compare them, as I said, to those animals that were living at the same time so we see if these humans are more like carnivores or herbivores of the site. And from that, we can conclude where most of their protein was coming from. So, we measure these in relation to other animals and we get an idea of the diet, of the lifetime diet of these hominids, these Neanderthals or modern humans."

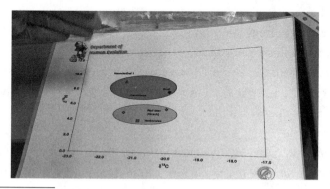

---

36 The Light Isotope Mass Spectrometry Laboratory (LIMSL) is a dedicated climate controlled laboratory that houses three stable isotope ratio mass spectrometers, and a variety of peripheral devices, for the analysis of light stable isotopes in both organic and inorganic material. The peripheral devices include a mass spectrometer interface for the measurement of compound specific isotopes such as amino acids.
*Edited from http://www.eva.mpg.de/evolution/files/isotopLab.htm

Smarter Hunters

At the time of our interview in 2006, this method of analysis[37] could look back over the last 100,000 years, which in Europe includes both the Neanderthals and our species of modern humans. Analysis of Neanderthals fossils identifies them as the top carnivores in the regions they inhabited, with all of their protein coming from animal sources. These findings are consistent throughout the entire period the Neanderthals walked the earth.

Around the time that Neanderthals began to disappear from the archaeological record in Europe, about 30,000 years ago, is also when the modern humans began dominating the landscape. When we compare Neanderthal food sources to modern humans' food sources, we see that the vast majority of it is the same—animal protein from medium to large herbivores. Modern humans, however, started showing a small portion of other proteins in their diet, from a broader range of food sources such as fish and smaller game. Perhaps this intentional broadening of their protein sources aided our species in harder, leaner times to come. The professor emphasized that this incorporation of new food sources by modern humans in Europe *"indicates a cognitive difference for our species too."* They had to develop new hunting strategies in order to go after these smaller kinds of resources.

The change from solely hunting large herbivores to including smaller food sources indicates our ancestors had started to think and live differently. One of my primary questions during these interviews is always this: does it make scientific sense as well as logical sense that we can learn things from their lifestyle that would then apply to us?

"I think so. If you think of this evolutionary trajectory... (how) modern humans got to be this way is over maybe 100,000 years of evolution, to get to the state of actually adapting to this diet. Of being a hunter-gatherer, moving around a lot, eating these wild foods. That's pretty clear. I think there's no question, that's what we really have adapted to be like."

---

37   They are constantly working on new technologies that can go back even further.

Carnivore or Omnivore?

One of the common assumptions about present day humans is that we are by nature "omnivores," often used to justify eating a plant centric diet. But "omnivore" defined really means "an animal or person that eats food of both animal and plant origin." Our ability to be omnivorous clearly doesn't automatically mean that it's ideal for us to eat mostly plants, and therefore we do not need significant amounts of animal foods in our diet.

Now that we have new information about human diet available, what *is* clear is this: whenever and wherever modern humans had the choice, we preferred animal foods. We get a lot more mileage out of eating a large horse or bison than gathering and eating plants, which are available only seasonally, especially in the parts of the world that went through the last great ice age. That severe climate change included much of Europe until about 10,000 years ago when the climate entered a warming cycle—the same warming cycle that we live in now. Also key to our survival is getting the critical nutrients from our diet that can only found in animal foods. Our species needed to have not only enough energy to survive, but also the right nutrients to thrive.

That said, Professor Richards believes that modern humans, even though we were top-level carnivores like Neanderthals, *can be* omnivorous, but as long as a choice was available, we chose meat. Then why eat plants? It's a survival strategy. We're not like some species that have only one kind of diet, or even one kind of food, and that if we divert from that diet, we die. We can adapt to dramatically changing circumstances and eat a range of diets and still survive when necessary. And even though this is not thriving, because we're able to utilize a broader range of foods, in anthropology, we are considered more "successful" as a species because of that ability.

"I think there's no question that for most of the time that we've been around, we had a nomadic lifestyle, with lots of exercise and eating a lot of animal protein and some wild plant foods. That's pretty clear."

Agriculture (for modern humans, a mixed bag)

This new technology also shows what happened to our species after we altered our primary source of protein from animal to plant sources.

"I spent a lot of time working on Neolithic and post-Neolithic sites as well, and there you really do see the humans with much lower nitrogen isotope values, and they are clearly getting a lot of the protein from plants."

The Neolithic (meaning "New Stone Age") is when agriculture has replaced the most recent Paleolithic (meaning "Old Stone Age") hunting lifestyle of modern humans.

When we were hunter-gatherers in Europe, it was a successful adaptation for about 30,000 years, but populations remained stable and very low. Before agriculture, the fossil evidence indicates that, outside of injuries and infections, we were strong, tall and healthy. After agriculture was introduced from the Near-East, you find a totally different situation. Populations grew, but people were shorter and had more cavities in their teeth. Their skeletons were weaker, less robust, and this universal decline in health is found everywhere agriculture was adopted. After agriculture began, there were also more and greater variety of diseases, diseases that followed a reduction in the quality of nutrition, and diseases from overcrowding due to the exploding population.

"So it's a bit of a trade-off, that you see. We're more successful, in a way, as a species, because there are more of us living in Europe...yet (have) shorter lives. You know, worse quality lifestyles...not as healthy (since agriculture)...There's a lot more people spreading out all over Europe and expanding like crazy in population."

Smart = Survival (then, *and* now)

Our transition from the hunter-gatherer lifestyle to living as farmers, beyond being successful in anthropological terms, created new and challenging problems for our species. We had become smarter, but was that newfound smart adaptability also the cause of our downfall in heath? As hunters, modern humans were always moving around, with some evidence for following reindeer herds in the early Paleolithic period. There is no evidence for real villages before agriculture.

At the very end of the Paleolithic period, just before agriculture, you start to see people living in groups, somewhat like villages. Especially along the coast where huge shell mounds show that we were just focusing in on one resource, like marine food. When these coastal humans' bone chemistry is analyzed, we can see they were eating nothing but fish and shellfish, and the professor explained that this is just a prelude to what happens next.

> "These people are probably ready for agriculture, which requires you to stay in one place. Because you just watch the crops, you watch the animals. And animal husbandry is the big thing in Europe for the first stages of agriculture. So you have to then change your lifestyle entirely. From being nomadic and moving around a lot, you have to start living in one place. By then, you have lot more food available. So, the population goes up. And this leads to villages and all the things we think of in the Neolithic[38] lifestyles."

Agriculture's Untold Secret
(my nutritional version of "The Devil is in the Details")

Agriculture started about 10,000 years ago and slowly moved from the Near East into southwestern Europe. Then about 5,000 years ago, there was a dramatic second wave that reached far north into new areas like Britain and Scandinavia. Let's use Britain to exemplify the part of the story that's missing for most of us.

Britain is interesting because it has broken away from the continent and become an island at this point. Up to now there is no evidence of agriculture, even when it was going on in Europe previously, until the second wave brought agriculture beyond the established (Neolithic) areas.

38 Neolithic is the "New Stone Age." Neo means New, Lithic means Stone.

After this new way of living reached Britain, you find people being buried in chamber tombs with pottery that wasn't there earlier.

From studying residues on some of the pottery from this period, there is good evidence that milk or cheese was being produced. You find animals and plants that were not in Britain before this, such as sheep and goats, along with domesticated cattle. These new animals had to be put on boats and brought to the island. We then see rapid change and adoption of this new lifestyle. Coinciding with this new lifestyle, there are more burials. These burial sites protected the bones, and Professor Richards has been able to measure the entire arc of food signatures from the bones of people living "old Stone Age" (Paleolithic) and "middle Stone Age" (Mesolithic) hunter-gatherer lifestyles from the same locations.

What he found was a truly remarkable change in diet and behavior. One example of this change is evidenced by the people who were buried on the coast. Their lifestyle was to collect and consume wild food exclusively from marine sources. This diet provided them all their needed proteins. After they were introduced to the Neolithic life, about 4,000 BC, Professor Richards was unable to find marine food signatures in the bones from these areas. It looks like they changed their way of life entirely, from gathering wild foods, to these new domesticated foods—meat and milk—that were easily available.

What's missing from the usual adoption of the agriculture story, and our subsequent decline in health, is that from the very beginning of this big change that these people *"still looked pretty healthy,"* Richards said, pointing to evidence. And here's why it's what I call Agriculture's Untold Secret.

Initially when the Neolithic arrived, these people were *not* interested in cereals (grains), but rather milk and domesticated meat. These early versions of domesticated animals and milk seem to have served them pretty well, more closely resembling the optimal nutritional profile of their previous wild foods, than the grain –based diet that was soon to come.

"At the beginning of the Neolithic there are a lot of places, where what they're interested in is not cereals, its milk and meat. Instead of hunting it, you can get it right there, because it's domesticated,"

Richards said. "And I imagine, for these people living in Britain, where all you've seen are these big aurochs, these massive wild cattle that are just huge, and all of a sudden you see these new Neolithic people have their own, a little bit smaller version of these; it had to be something… I think that's what is behind the main spread of the last phase of the Neolithic in northern Europe. I think it was animal protein that people were going for."

Only later when more and more cereals were introduced do we start to see cavities in their teeth from too much carbohydrate, their stature dropping, their skeletons becoming weaker and less robust.

Vegetarians and the Archaeological Record

While talking with the professor about plant foods, becoming modern humans and our main sources of protein, I wondered if, prior to agriculture, there were any modern human vegetarians.

"I really don't think so. And it's extremely hard to find vegetarians, even archaeologically. In all the studies, we measured thousands and thousands of humans from all over the world; I think we have yet to find a vegetarian or a vegan. … Sometimes we do, but we go back and realize that (the archaeologist) actually sampled a cow or something, by mistake. I don't think I've ever seen anyone who would be a vegan (before agriculture), ever."

Professor Richards noted that a modern human living as a vegetarian in those times would not have just been difficult, *"I think it would be epically impossible."* He said, *"You can't really survive that way. The only way we could survive just on plants (grains) is if you can process them."* What that means is that you would have to take them and turn them into cereals, bread or porridges to make their protein accessible.

If you were going to be vegetarian and lived in some parts of northern Europe, during a short period called the Mesolithic or "Middle Stone Age," just before agriculture and the "New Stone Age" fully takes over, you might have been able to find an abundance of hazelnuts in order to survive. Big pits full of burnt hazelnut shells have been uncovered. Modern humans could get a lot of protein out of them and *"survive quite well on that,"* Richards said. But the trouble is, like all plant foods, that food source option is seasonal. You couldn't survive the rest of the year just being vegetarian.

Additionally, part of the survival equation for our species, is that the food we eat must provide all of the essential nutrients needed to be our healthiest and to thrive.

> *"There are crucial, key things that humans need to survive. There are essential amino acids and fatty acids that without them your brains aren't going to develop when you're a child. Without these proteins you will not lay down new muscle…your heart and all these muscles are always turning over. Without the proteins, without these amino acids you'll die. I mean, you can't do it."*

Our bones, our bodies, are continuously "turning over" protein, which is a continuous process of forming new cells and reabsorbing old cells. So even as you're reading this book, collagen is leaving your bones and new collagen has been made to go in. The amino acids that are being used for that are from that what you ate for breakfast or lunch, depending on the time of day. Whatever protein you had, that is now going into your bone collagen.

When the professor tests a bone, the results show what's happened over that individual's life. He's getting this picture of all the protein, if you can imagine, that's been eaten over 20, 30, 40 years. So it's a broad measure of diet. But it's extremely powerful, because it tells us what people were doing day-to-day, over their lifetimes.

> *"It's really sampling all the time through life, every kind of meal and the kind of protein. We can get a picture of their overall lifetime diet. So, short-term subtleties, we wouldn't see if Neanderthals ate plants for one week. I don't think we would see it. We really are looking*

at the big picture. And one of the really big pictures is that animal proteins were the main dietary source for Neanderthals (and modern humans). And for these modern humans to have a signal that shows fish, maybe 20 - 25%. That means, effectively, a quarter of the year, or every third or fourth meal, would be fish. So, it's a very broad tool, but very powerful, as well."

The current wide-ranging adoption of grain and plant based foods in westernized countries might be regarded as "a new evolutionary experiment." For most of modern humans, this kind of eating has only dominated our diet for, at most, the last 5,000 years out of a time spanning over more than 100,000 years. Now, faced with an exploding food-induced international health crisis, the growing epidemic of obesity and diet-related chronic inflammatory diseases, many of us are desperately looking for the best way to fix it.

So what's the answer? Using the hard scientific facts of what was once unknowable we can now identify the authentic food sources on which modern humans thrived. We can relearn from the last 100,000 years what we knew when we were our strongest and healthiest, enabling us to once again achieve that high level of good health.

"If you think of it that way, what we are adapted to is not what we are living right now," Richards said "This kind of Paleolithic diet (not current popular "paleo" diets [39])... it's probably the most optimum for modern humans. It has to be. It's what evolutionary pressures pushed us towards, and we were successful in that kind of diet...It's got to be the best diet for humans."

---

39 Author emphasis.

Reporter's Notebook

Authentic Human Diet: Tech Breakthrough
1. Exactly what modern humans ate on a regular basis, sites worldwide.
2. Diets of animals and Neanderthals who lived in these sites.
3. Exactly what modern humans ate when health began to decline.
4. Essential source of information could help solve major health problems we face today.

Humans:
1. Top-level carnivores like Neanderthals.
2. "Can be" omnivorous as survival strategy.
3. As long as a choice was available, we chose meat.

Agriculture:
1. A mixed bag.
2. Populations grew, but people were shorter, more cavities in teeth.
3. Skeletons weaker, less robust.
4. Universal decline in health found everywhere agriculture adopted.
5. Greater variety of diseases followed this reduction in quality of nutrition.
6. Also, diseases from overcrowding due to exploding population.

Adoption:
1. Started in Near East approx. 10k yrs. ago.
2. Slowly moved into Southwestern Europe.
3. 5k yrs. ago dramatic second wave carries into Briton & Scandinavia.

The Untold Secret:

1. At beginning of change people still looked pretty healthy.
2. Why: people not interested in cereals (grains), but rather milk and domesticated meat.
3. Early versions of domesticated animals and milk more closely resembled the optimal nutritional profile of previous wild foods than the grain - based diet.
4. Animal protein is what people were going for.

Pre-Agriculture:

1. No vegetarians or vegans found in archeological record.
2. Crucial, key things that humans need to survive.
3. Living as vegetarian in those times not just difficult, but *"epically impossible."*

The Bottom Line... *With new technology we can see the big picture. The main dietary source of protein for Neanderthals and modern humans was animal protein.*

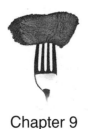

THINK PROVEN:
THE NEW MEDICINE

Chapter 9

"Well, the motivator comes, I think, from the diet itself... It's very self-perpetuating. Once you've gotten on it, you feel so much better, and most people say that "I don't know if I've ever felt this good."

"Also, when you've been on the diet for a while and you go off the diet, it's like your body reminds you, no, that's not human food, and it steers you right back on. You can end up with some negative effects, very profound, from eating foods that you're not supposed to be eating."

—**Lane Sebring, MD**, To C.J. Hunt in
The Perfect Human Diet documentary

A fter Professor Richards said this way of eating has got to be *"the best diet for humans"* I wanted to understand the practical applications. In other words, how we could all use this game changing knowledge today in our modern world, with the foods and resources available to us now to proactively create the health and life we deserve.

I called Professor Cordain[40] to see what kind of user results he could share with me from his research into human nutrition. He told me, while it was true that he was receiving lots of enthusiastic email from people who had followed his recommendations and improved their health, his specialty was research as an academic, not as a medical practitioner treating patients. Those happy emails he had received were personal accounts, anecdotal accounts, rather than scientific facts or rigorous clinical research. But, he *did* know of a medical professional who was putting the human evolutionary nutrition method of eating into practice with real patients and, as he put it, had *"converted half the town!"* He was telling me about Dr. Lane Sebring of the Sebring Clinic in Wimberley, Texas.

Not only was Dr. Sebring the very first U.S. medical doctor to fully embrace the evolution-based eating principles in his practice, he was having *"extraordinary results with his patients."* And just as importantly for a journalist such as myself, he had kept extensive patient records that documented these life-changing transformations since day one.

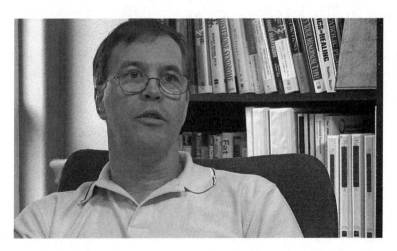

---

40   The Paleo Diet: Lose Weight and Get Healthy by Eating the Food You Were
      Designed to Eat Hardcover – December 7, 2001 by Loren Cordain, PhD.

Dr. Lane Sebring is the founding physician of the Sebring Clinic and is a recognized expert in Alternative and Anti-Aging Medicine. He has built a unique reputation for helping patients for whom modern medicine has failed. He endeavors to eliminate or at least reduce patients' prescription drugs using natural methods of healing that *"respect their bodies' original design."*

After spending a day filming at the clinic, I would say he's much more than what can be seen on his extensive professional credentials. I found him to be more like the idealized version of doctors I remember from late1950s and early 60s when I was growing up, how they took as much time as needed to care for their patients, not rushing through as many as possible each hour. In addition to what one would expect in an initial medical evaluation with a physician, Dr. Sebring devotes extra time to teach his patients about the nature of disease, how to avoid it, and how the right diet can reverse and heal disease. Dietary changes that will maximize their functionality at a high level throughout the rest of their lives.

Dr. Sebring explained to me that when a new patient starts under his care, part of the first visit is *"an initial 45 minute lecture"* (My first exposure to his dry, Texas hill country, sense of humor). That "45 minute lecture" is really the focused one-on-one opportunity to cover the most important points he would like his patients to understand as they substantially upgrade their personal commitment to their own health.

"The most important thing they need to know is that they can take control of their health, that they don't need to be dependent on the drug companies, that they can avoid the need for that. And they do that by diet... we are what we eat. That's an old cliché, but it's absolutely true. The problem is, before now, we didn't know what to eat. We used to know, thousands of years ago; it was handed down, what was a smart thing to eat. But now we don't, because we're told by industry and not by our great-great grandparents. It's not been handed down. So we're off-track, and that's the message I try to get to my patients. They can be in control. All these diseases that we see, all these chronic problems, virtually every one of them are eliminated by

a good diet. Evidence is there to support that. My patients prove it. So I try to get that across."

Respecting Natures Design

Dr. Sebring's personal journey into human evolutionary nutrition—and making it the foundation of his practice—was pretty straightforward, once he was exposed to the information. He defines himself as a conceptual thinker, and with this evolutionary method of eating, all of the pieces fit *"the big picture"* - he couldn't find any contradiction.

> *"It wasn't contrary to anything that I knew. It really fit. It explained it. I may have to look at it a little bit differently, but once you explained it, it all made great sense. For me, I thought, this fits with my philosophy of life. I may be a bit of a romanticist about man having come from nature, but nonetheless, it really fits. And simply, following from that, health improves. It's consistent."*

It soon became clear to me that he thoroughly enjoys teaching these principles. During portions of the interview when I normally am the one who's asking the most questions he took over like I was a new patient, and it became this journalists "45 minute lecture."

Dr. Sebring: *"Wild animals are healthy; you ever see a wild animal overweight?"*

Hunt: "No."

Dr. Sebring: *"Why? Because they're eating the foods they were designed to eat."*

Hunt: "Are they a lot more active than we are?"

Dr. Sebring: *"When you observe hunter-gatherers they are active people, but their workday is 2 1/2 hours… And yet, they are not overweight.*

One of the important things missing from our conventional perspective on diet is that we are predators. If you go looking for *true* hunter-gatherers, it becomes difficult to use them as the example because there are very few left.

Hunt: "Have you seen any accurate depictions of true hunter-gatherers on television?"

Dr. Sebring: *"Most of the hunter-gatherers you see on television have been marginalized off their lands, and have been forced to grow something six months out of the year, or so. They're not nearly as healthy as those who are still doing pure hunting and gathering. If you find true hunter-gatherers, the men have got six-packs, and the women have their feminine shape, but nobody's overweight and nobody's underweight. They're strong; they're very powerful people."*

Hunt: "Those that are still the native hunter-gatherers?"

Sebring: *"Right. Those that are still the native hunter-gatherers. You know, look at most of your old pictures of Eskimos, the Inuit Indian and his Inuit Indian wife, and there's nothing but blue sky for background and big smiles. I think it's the omega-three's (needed for optimal brain function), I am pretty convinced of that. It's what they get from their diet.*

You've got to have the big picture; you have to back off and look at it. And that's what looking at life on earth does when you go back and look at hunter-gatherers. It's a much bigger picture. Instead of trying to tease out what causes this disease and what causes that disease. Looking at this picture, we didn't used to have all these problems. What was different? Well, the answer is that the same causes exist for all of them, and its diet.

It's ironic that, as a scientist, you expect science to pull us through. But science is so focused, it often misses the big picture. I often think of it (science) as on the left side of the brain. It's very narrow, linear type of logic. But the right side of the brain has a very big picture focus. We sort of ignore that. Left-

brain thinking says, "Concepts are cute, but what are you going to do with that? You've got to prove the ground you stand on."

But if that's the direction you're going, you can't see when you've gotten off the pathway to health, or anything else."

Obesity and Diet-Related Chronic Disease

Dr. Sebring is a practitioner who works with patients every day. As such, I was particularly interested in what his feelings were about the big health problems dominating the news, as well as his work with individual patients. Problems like:

1. The obesity epidemic, which in the United States kills nearly 400,000 people a year.
2. Diet-induced chronic inflammatory diseases.
3. If our genetics predispose us to disease no matter what we do.
4. And, the current U.S.D.A. Food Plate recommendations (updated from the well-known food pyramid).

Because, like every physician, he had started right out of medical school practicing conventional medicine, Dr. Sebring had years of clinical experience seeing what kinds of results that standard medical approach produced for his patients. But now, looking at the obesity epidemic with the knowledge he's gained from the evolutionary diet guidelines he's put into practice with his patients, and seeing "the very positive results", it evokes a strong heartfelt reaction witnessing so many overweight and obese people worldwide unknowingly make bad dietary choices.

"From my position, now, I find that seeing that (the obesity epidemic)… it's not only painful, it's also frustrating. Because I feel that if we can get the message out of what we need to do about it, that we can avoid that. Or, at least, we can empower people to make the choice. They don't know what choices to make now. And if we can educate them, so that they, at least, know they're making the wrong choice if they decide to do that, then I think we've done something.

But I think that most people will choose to correct their problems on the downhill course that we're currently on. "

Chronic Inflammatory Disease

In addition to the obesity epidemic, another big part of the downhill course we're currently on includes the many chronic inflammatory diseases that are diet induced. Diseases like rheumatoid arthritis, Alzheimer's, Graves' disease, multiple sclerosis and more. For example, the *National Institute of Arthritis and Musculoskeletal and Skin Diseases* (NIAMS), a part of the *U.S. Department of Health and Human Services' National Institutes of Health* (NIH), says:

> *"Autoimmune diseases can affect almost any part of the body, including the heart, brain, nerves, muscles, skin, eyes, joints, lungs, kidneys, glands, the digestive tract, and blood vessels. In an autoimmune reaction, antibodies and immune cells target the body's own healthy tissues by mistake, signaling the body to attack them."*[41]

And like the obesity epidemic, according to NAIMS director Stephen I. Katz, M.D., Ph.D., it affects thousands of lives; *"Almost every household in America is affected in some way by diseases of bones, joints, muscles, and skin."*

Dr. Sebring explained to me how inflammatory disease works. The major cause for all autoimmune diseases is undigested proteins getting into the bloodstream; the body sees that undigested protein as an antigen (a toxin or other foreign substance), and in an effort to protect the body, attacks it. Then, somewhere else in the body our immune system sees a molecule that looks like that protein and begins to attack it. A more specific example would be Bacteroides, which *is* a very common gut bacterium. If it gets presented to the immune system because of a leaky inflamed gut, generally caused by grains, then the immune system sees that bacteria as an invader and attacks it. Some people, because of their genetics, have protein

---

41   http://www.niams.nih.gov/HEALTH_INFO/Autoimmune/default.asp

in their joint cartilage that looks exactly like Bacteroides. So not only is the body attacking this protein from the bacteria's cell wall where it is needed, but it also starts attacking the cartilage in their joints. For these people, this is the onset of rheumatoid arthritis.

Disease: Genetics or Environment

We are often told that these inflammatory chronic diseases (and other diseases) are genetic, inevitable no matter what we do. The conventional treatment, if any exists for that particular inflammatory disease, is pharmaceutical, often in the form of over-the-counter anti-inflammatories, like ibuprofen (e.g. Motrin, Advil) or stronger versions available only by prescription, and even steroids. Of course now medicine acknowledges that using those on a regular basis can be harmful, recommending minimal dosages for restricted periods.

An important question to ask about inflammatory and chronic disease is this: is rheumatoid arthritis genetic and therefore "inevitable" or is it environmental? The answer is something most of us have never heard before and is one of those concepts that require us to "think differently" because the answer is *"yes… it's both."*

Dr. Sebring tells his patients to think of it like this: if you're living in the Garden of Eden, if you're living in that environment from which we came, all those genes fit. Some families have more reserve capacity in certain metabolic pathways in the body, chemical pathways, than do other families. But in both of these families, that additional reserve capacity doesn't get used up in that environment. Everyone has all the reserve required to handle the stresses that can happen in that ideal environment. Come out of that environment into our modern, crowded, stress-filled and polluted world, and sometimes, those metabolic pathways are required to handle ten, twenty, even a hundred times more activity, and they are not able to handle that. They can't do that. And some families, in particular, just cannot.

"It manifests as symptoms of disease. And we say, "Ah, it's genetic!"
Modern medicine is like this: "Ah, you've got high cholesterol. Runs

in your family, doesn't it? Yes, it's genetic. Here's some Lipitor." Now you're married to the pharmaceutical industry for the rest of your life.... But the problem is (in our natural environments) normal cholesterol is 120;[42] *the healthy range is 100 to 140. Where's genetics? We're talking about people from the Poles, to the equator, to the remote Sea Islands. You couldn't find a more genetically diverse group. Yet, they all have excellent cholesterol. So, again, genetics is important only in the context of a bad diet."*

In our modern world we've changed so many things and created so many new stressors that there are many more threats to our health and well-being. From what the doctor was telling me, we're really designed for very low stress and now we're getting stressors that are way outside of our design limits. An analogy would be, in our modern world we can easily handle a steady state of 20% stressors. With a strong reserve from following a good diet and active lifestyle we can handle additional stressors that climb to 100%. We can even survive if it gets to 120% for a short period of time. But now we're often way beyond our capacity on a daily basis.

"Sometimes I feel like we're on the precipice here of falling off. Maybe, we've learned just enough, just in time…that we can grab ourselves before we fall off the precipice of health here, and it's going fast. Nobody's paying attention. Everybody has their individual plan for themselves, basically, to perpetuate their wealth or what have you, instead of looking at the big picture. They're not thinking about their kids or grandkids. Nutritionists now often say that the kids born today

---

42   "A total cholesterol of 122 sounds very low, particularly in a country like the U.S. where the norm is 206, but in nature, a total cholesterol of 122 is the rule. The total cholesterol of primates like chimpanzees ranges from 110 to 140, as does the total cholesterol of primitive hunter-gatherers living today – and neither primates nor hunter-gatherers have heart attacks. By every line of evidence, having a total cholesterol value below 130, or certainly below 150, is ideal for avoiding heart disease." Source: *What Do My Cholesterol Numbers Mean?* (https://www.pritikin. com/your-health/health-benefits/lower-cholesterol/783-what-do-my-cholesterol-numbers-mean.html)

will not outlive their parents, because they never had good nutrition. I've got eleven year-old type II diabetics, dietary-induced diabetes. And when I first graduated medical school I never saw anybody under 55 with type-II diabetes. I've got children that haven't even hit puberty yet and they've got type-II diabetes. So, we've made a lot of mistakes. Hopefully, we can turn this around."

USDA Food Pyramid:[43] *Good Advice or Bad*?

In 2006 when I asked Dr. Sebring about the USDA's Food Pyramid nutritional guidance (renamed *the Food Plate*), if it's good or bad advice, he said, *"It depends on who is making the assessment. If it's the agricultural industry (plant agriculture: grains, corn, soy, etc.), it's a great idea, except they're not thinking long-term because they're killing their patrons."* Explaining further he said the food pyramid, if you look at the proportions of the carbs and proteins and fats, is exactly the same that we use to fatten our hogs. So it should be no surprise that our weight keeps going up. To me the clear follow-up question was, *"If following the food pyramid recommendations puts our health seriously at risk, and you had the opportunity to rebuild it, what would you do? What would it look like?"* That question launched the doctor into another of his many fascinating stories.

He told me he had once heard a lecture from a very intelligent physician who was talking about this very thing. His food pyramid started with water. "It was a floating pyramid," the lecturing physician said. And Dr. Sebring agrees with that—water would be the base of this new healthy pyramid.

"People ask me on this human food diet, "but doc, what do I drink?" Well, try water. It's hard for some people to do that, but once you do that and you've been doing that for a while, that's what you want. It's

---

43   In 2006 at the time of the interview the government advice was still promoted as the USDA food pyramid. Since that time it has gone through one change has now called the "food plate." these recommendations are reviewed every five years and the next version will come out in 2015.

hard to change the old habits, but, again, the diet, it self-perpetuates; it's what you crave. And so, I would start with water."

After that, the next level of that new pyramid would be protein. So outside of drinking plenty of water every day, each meal should start with *"a major source of protein."* Next up would be non-starchy vegetables (vegetables that grow above the ground). Surround that major source of protein with all the vegetables that you want. You can add some additional healthy fats, particularly if you've chosen a lean protein or want to dress up your vegetables a bit (healthy fats are defined in Chapter 10). Then topping off the pyramid would be small amounts of low sugar fruits such as berries, and nuts, which you could have with the meal; and *"they work great for snacks in between meals as well".*

The Body Wants to Heal

One of Dr. Sebring's friends brought him a syllabus from a conference he had attended where one of the speakers was a neurologist. The speaker referred to another neurologist from back in the 30s or 40s that was a specialist in multiple sclerosis. That neurologist had put a lot of his patients on a special diet to help them improve their health, and he followed about 80 patients for several decades. He said there was virtually no progression of their MS for the people that went on this special diet. And the diet consisted of all the non-starchy vegetables; fruits and nuts; the lean meats — chicken, fish, turkey; effectively, they cut out grains, dairy, beans and potatoes.

"Basically the same dietary recommendations I use," said Dr. Sebring. Several of his patients with MS have been on the human food diet and they've been holding steady for a long time. *"They get an initial improvement by going on the diet, and some still have an occasional flare up, but they're maintaining steady… and most importantly, are not in decline."* One patient had an MRI of her brain with such surprising results the neurologist called Dr. Sebring to share some unexpected news: *"She had lesions there, on her brain, that are completely gone now!"*

For us, the great news here is that the body wants to heal. When you give your body what it needs, when you give a cell what it needs to perform a function, it wants to heal. But today in our modern world we keep short circuiting it by feeding it *"poisonous foods that are toxic to the body."* Dr. Sebring said, *"We have the capacity to heal. We didn't think the brain could heal. But now we find out in the last few years that it has stem cells that can heal the brain."*

When Dr. Sebring was in medical school, he and his classmates were taught that cartilage couldn't regenerate; it just wears out. But now, we know that's not true.

"How does anything last for 100 years? Of course, it can repair. And the body can repair. And that's the good news. When you get the nutrition the body needs, a lot of problems go away you didn't know were problems. A lot of people say, "So that's how that's supposed to work, I see now," because their body is functioning much better and they don't have those problems. Life isn't supposed to be this hard. Hunter-gatherers have a rather exposed lifestyle, certainly from what we typically experience, but I think their overall health was far superior… and maybe their ultimate enjoyment was, also."

The opportunity to regenerate and heal our body can restore our hope as well. One of the things Dr. Sebring tells his patients is that it's nice to know improvement is possible.

"At some point in your life you don't believe that anymore. Every year, the doctor adds a new pill to your list, and you've got a new problem, and whether real or perceived, it's how you feel, what you think is going on. And the hope starts to fade. And this (diet) puts their health back into their hands and they can start pulling off pills. You should be monitored by a doctor, I have to throw that in, but it happens… it happens routinely."

Take Charge

Of course, to prevent or reverse disease, one of the biggest parts of improving our health is personally taking charge of the things we can control, like our daily diet. His patients are very encouraged that they can do this sort of thing and they can improve, that so much more control of their health is in their own hands. By all indications there are more and more people willing to take on that responsibility now.

"People are very frustrated with the way things are going, they see this isn't right, something is wrong. Most people, on some level, recognize that we're out of sync here. We don't have room for our wisdom teeth. What's wrong with that? And paleo explains all that to them. So they begin to say "this makes sense.""

Unfortunately, at this point in time if we go to a conventional doctor for care and ask them about evolutionary health and this kind of dietary change, the whole thing is brushed aside as being nonsense. In fact, the *American Diabetes Association* still recommends a high carbohydrate, low fat, low protein diet for diabetics.[44] The ADA's current 2014 published guidelines say "no one-size-fits-all", that you should see an advisor or practitioner to guide you. But upon examination these guidelines are effectively the same as the old USDA Food Pyramid, saying *"To ensure you eat healthfully your focus should be on whole grains, fruits, vegetables, beans and low-fat milk..."* Dr. Sebring's thoughts on the issue are clear:

"That's insane. They (the patients) are guaranteed to be ending up on insulin, and perpetuating the drugs that we give."

He also understands how that thinking has evolved. Not long ago the only way physicians had to treat diabetes, besides diet (the original tool), was to add in insulin. The biggest problem a doctor had, his biggest fear,

---

44   To guide you their first recommendation is a Registered Dietitian. In order to remain part of their organization, the Academy of Nutrition and Dietetics, they *must* use the organizations official guidelines, currently the USDA Food Plate.

was that his patient was going to have a low blood sugar in the middle of the night. So the prescription was to eat small meals throughout the day (still the same in 2014) and keep your carbs up, because they don't want you to have low blood sugar.

> *"That's how we got this high carbohydrate thing going. And then, the high carbohydrates and the high insulin levels destroyed the kidneys… so then we would say that protein's tough on the kidneys. Yeah, at the very last minute, before you go over the edge, it can be a little tough on a patient, so then we say cut back on the proteins…but (it will take time to correct this idea), it takes 50 years for a paradigm shift after new knowledge is available."*

Conventional Medicine: *Change Happens, Slowly*

As an example, Dr. Sebring told me a story about Max Planck, the father of quantum physics. Dr. Planck showed us that our planetary model of the atom, with electrons traveling around it like planets around the sun, was not accurate. He had very compelling evidence but he was crucified by his peers. *"Don't tell me, I've been teaching this for 25 years, I've got evidence, myself!"* they would say. He was interviewed a few years after he had published these papers, and was asked, *"Tell us Dr. Planck, how do you see science advancing?"* He replied, *"Funeral by funeral."*

> *"That's kind of harsh, but you can certainly see his sentiment and identify with that, looking at the way (those) things are going on. And if you don't shake those people, or don't push them aside, our experts, push them aside and look at the evidence yourself for the human food and the non-human foods way of thinking about this…we're going to continue in the direction that we're going and it won't get better; it's going to get worse. Everything you can see points to that."*

Hunt: "The way that I've heard that, and usually it's in other contexts, and it seems to fit here, is that if you keep going the way you're going, you're liable to end up where you were headed."

Sebring: *"That's right. Another way of saying it is if you don't do anything different, don't expect anything different to happen."*

Hunt: "Right, the definition of insanity, doing the same thing and expecting a different outcome."

Sebring: *"Which describes us now."*

USDA Food Plate: *A New Look for Old Thinking*

Today, as has been the advice of the Food Pyramid (now Food Plate) since the 1960's, most people rely on carbohydrates from non-human foods; grains, starches (from tubers and potatoes), packaged refined foods made from these, and refined sugars, to form glucose in order to supply energy to their cells. Eating these type of carbohydrates is like stoking your body's fire with small twigs of kindling wood. You'll get a quick flash of fire that burns quickly. You'll get some quick energy, but it doesn't sustain you. The alternative, when you fuel your fire with healthy proteins and fats, is like throwing a slow burning log on your body's fire that will keep giving you a steady flame (energy) for hours.

Dr. Sebring tries to get patients to realize that they should think about protein foods as being *time-released* glucose[45] (blood sugar). The liver can take these protein foods and turn them into glucose in a time-released fashion. When you work harder and you need more energy, your body makes more glucose from these healthy animal foods. *"That's how we're truly designed. How beautiful is that? So you have steady energy all day long."*

But if you choose to eat a bunch of non-human food carbohydrates, stoke your fire with kindling wood, then your insulin level goes up. That

---

45   Glucose is the main type of sugar in the blood and is (believed to be) the major source of energy for the body's cells. Glucose comes from the foods we eat or the body can make it from other substances. Glucose is carried to the cells through the bloodstream. Several hormones, including insulin, control glucose levels in the blood. Source http://kidshealth.org/parent/diabetes_center/words_know/glucose.html

insulin goes to your liver, and once there shuts off the conversion of proteins into glucose. So now, if you had protein for breakfast, you shut off your body's ability to burn that protein for energy.

"Your systems are going to start crashing pretty soon, and at that point, the only way to get it back up (your blood sugar) is either to rest a little bit… or you can stuff more protein in and that will bring it back up. But a lot of times, at that point, they are craving carbs. They want something quick and they want it now. "I don't feel good!" And that's what we see. You should think of proteins as setting the thermostat to 72 degrees, and then go (on with your day)."

"Quality of Life" Extension

Dr. Sebring went on to tell me another quick story about a fellow who did autopsies on people who lived to be over 100, and that his observations about them were very good. The coroner looked at them and said, *"You know, these people had all the problems of aging, they have them all. But, everything got old evenly."* And that, said Dr. Sebring, was a brilliant conclusion. That's the way we should age.

"After 30, you don't heal as fast, and you're going, what's up with that? And by 40, you're going to need glasses, etc. So it seems like it's my responsibility, as a physician, to find out if someone has a weak system and if that's the case, we can support it, so everything gets old evenly."

That story illustrates another important advantage to eating the human food diet; it helps everything get old evenly. It helps us to maintain our functionality over a much longer period of time. Then there's an accelerated aging at the end of life. It's not the long downhill decline most people in industrialized countries have come to expect that eats away at our dignity. It may not extend ultimate life expectancy, but more people will get to their ultimate maximum age. And then, accelerated aging at the end. Just like we see in nature.

"I often tell people that I want to be found dead, in the garden, at some age over 100, with a flower in my hand and pollen on my nose. That's sort of ideal. But maintaining the functionality is what we're looking for."

An intriguing example he shared is about some hunter-gatherer groups in the Venezuelan jungle. There, a young man often has more than one wife in his lifetime because he gets married the first time when he's 13 or 14, and his first wife is usually around 60.

"Now, what does that tell you about the health of 60-year-old hunter-gatherer women? They're maintaining their functionality. They have to, to keep up. And that's what happens when you eat what humans were designed to eat."

Big Healthy Brains

The doctor explained that when our species started eating meats that allowed the brain to double in size. *"Over 25% of our energy is used in the brain"*, and he's seen studies that the energy use is as high as 70%, depending on what factors they're looking at. Emphasizing, it's important to understand that we had this compact source of food that was animal protein and fats that are very nutrient-dense, and that then allowed us to double our brain size.

"We don't want to forsake that; there is a reason why it worked that way... And when we do (forsake that), we get into trouble."

Ambiguity: *The Achilles Heel of current "Paleo" Diets*

Now that I had met with the leading anthropologists in the field of human evolutionary nutrition, and witnessed the innovative scientific technology that reveals the authentic human diet with Mike Richards at the *Max Planck Institute of Evolutionary Anthropology*, I was keen to hear what Dr. Sebring had done with the original paleo diet ideas to make them more effective. I was particularly interested because there continues to be growing public confusion around what "paleo" means and what foods are honestly "paleo," due to many enthusiasts—and the media—putting their own spins on it. Along with an astounding amount of business opportunists riding the current wave of paleo's popularity who are willing to label just about anything as "paleo." We spoke briefly about the growing confusion around the Paleo diet concept, which in the last couple of years has rapidly accelerated. Dr. Sebring said this the underlying problem:

> *"People try to squeeze their favorite foods into it and still call it "paleo" — but it's not."*

For example, pick up any diet or cookbook book in your local Barnes & Noble with "paleo" in the title and each book includes foods the other doesn't. And it's no different on the Internet. Easy to understand how this can be confusing, especially to people just exploring the idea for the first time. Dr. Sebring's position as a physician is clear. If there are enthusiasts and authors who want to incorporate some of the principles, while also adding to or tinkering with the original researched based paleo food list, that's fine, *"but they shouldn't label it "paleo.""*

To date, the rapidly popularized paleo diet's core group of enthusiasts and promoters has been younger, highly athletic, technologically savvy, relatively healthy populations; millennials with some overlap into Gen-X'rs.[46] Their big drivers are weight loss, looking great, athletic performance and better health, better sex and connecting socially with other enthusiasts, easy to do now thanks to the Internet.

As the first practicing physician to fully embrace the original[47] Paleolithic diet concepts, Dr. Sebring's patients have primarily sought him

---

46 1964-82 Gen-X, Researchers and commentators use birth years ranging from the early 1980s to the early 2000s. http://en.wikipedia.org/wiki/Millennials

47 *The Paleo Diet*, Loren Cordain, PhD. Wiley, December 2001.

out not to improve athletic performance or to lose weight, but to reclaim their health; and from that, a much better life. Conventional medicine, or their personal attempts to follow what they had been told was "a healthy diet," had failed them. When they first walked in the front door of the clinic they simply wanted to feel better. And for those that became devotees of what they discovered by walking through those doors, many achieved remarkably outstanding results; results they could never have imagined when they first walked in.

Dr. Sebring's practice effectively became "paleo ground zero," the first testing ground to discover what worked, and what didn't work, from those original guidelines in a medical practice. And also safely engage patient's incorporation of appropriate supplementation and other natural methods to improve the results his patients received.

Given the unfortunate reality that the word "paleo" *has* been co-opted[48] by so many, and the growing public confusion stemming from these variations, I asked if it might be better to call the diet something else? Like an "ideal diet"? Make it more user friendly to anyone seeking a healthier and happier life. With some luck, repositioning it with better language to make it less academic and more personal might also eventually influence the media to be more accurate, rather than continually mocking it as "the caveman diet" in order to question its relevancy to us now.

The Confusion Solution: *Smart Innovation*

As a broadcast journalist, scientific accuracy, relevancy and viewer accessibility is why I gave the film its working title during production as *In Search of the Perfect Human Diet*, and then in distribution as simply *The Perfect Human Diet*.

Dr. Sebring still uses the word "Paleo" in public talks, in the name of his nutritional supplement "pharmacy" which adjoins the clinic (The Paleo Pharmacy), or when first introducing the diet to patients. But the down to earth language he then uses to help his patients understand and use

---

48   Divert to or use in a role different from the usual or original one.

the concepts came as a pleasant surprise to me with his use of the words "human" and "non-human."

It's not hard to imagine that Albert Einstein would have loved this smart and practical hard science based innovation to help solve the public confusion about the many published "paleo" diets, or any other dietary confusion for that matter. As you'll see here, and next in Chapter 10, it fits Professor Einstein's idea perfectly, *"No idea is so complex that it can't be explained simply."*

The Next Wave in Diet & Health: *The Perfect Human Diet*

> *"For my patient's sake, and in some ways for myself, I sort of break food into two categories: human food, and non-human food. And the human foods would be: the lean meats, turkey, fish, chicken... preferably from an animal that was eating what it was designed to eat... fruits, nuts and vegetables.*
>
> *The non-human foods would be: the grains, which is probably the worst problem that we have; dairy, after two years old; we're not designed for dairy after two years old, certainly not from another animal; and beans and potatoes.*
>
> *And so, those are the simple categories that I put them in, and people understand that, I understand that, and it helps me to make choices."*

Using Dr. Sebring's categories, starting with non-human foods, I asked him "What's wrong with grains?" He answered, beginning with the clarification that we can approach that question from many different directions. One, the archaeological record is quite crystal-clear. Grains caused us to lose height. Grain consumption caused a narrowing of the sphenoid bone (situated in the middle of the skull towards the front), which is now not strong enough to support the full weight and buttress the skull. The result

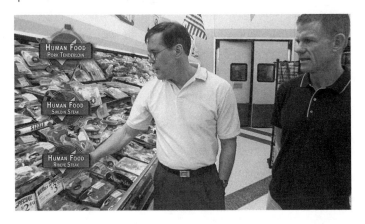

is that we now have smaller brains as a consequence of eating grains. *"We have more scrunched up noses we can't breathe through. And we have a jaw that can't hold a full complement of teeth, and so we have overlapping teeth; we have no room for our wisdom teeth."* These negative effects are common to all civilized groups on the planet following the introduction of grains into their diet.

> *"Grains block the absorption of magnesium; if you can't absorb magnesium, you can't absorb calcium. Grains bind up our digestive enzymes. They bring in gluten, they bring in yeast; they cause a chronic inflammatory state of the gut and is a big initiator of almost all of our chronic inflammatory diseases— autoimmune diseases, rheumatoid arthritis—virtually absent in the archeological record, prior to the institution of grains into the diet."*

I found it interesting too that there is a "most harmful" hierarchy to that list of non-human foods Dr. Sebring defined. In his clinical experience, grains are the most important to take out of the diet. There are a few people that may have an allergy to a particular food, but as a group, grains are by far the most important to take out of the diet. He also told me the exact reasons as to why were still being investigated, but present statistical analysis shows if you introduce grains to a baby in the first three months of life, that child is 8 to 12 times more likely to end up as a child diabetic. Even the introduction of grains within the first six months or year contributes greatly to the onset of diabetes sometime in life.

Think Doctor Proven (and more user friendly)

His clinical experience also shows him that to refer to the foods commonly available to us, the foodstuffs most of us have been raised on as "human food and non-human food" works very well, and helps patients stay on track.

> *"I think it fits; I think it's appropriate. Starvation foods (grains, dairy, beans and potatoes) are not the choices we need to be making unless we're under starvation. I mean, maybe we're on a planet under starvation food mode. And so there we are, we're all having to eat grains to stay alive. If you're in a situation where you're starving, then go ahead and eat these foods. But if you're not starving, there's no need to eat these foods. You get everything you need in glorious abundance when you have the fruits and nuts and vegetables and the lean animal protein and the fats that are there from a healthy animal...the fats are very good for you."*

When it comes to "human foods," that list starts with animal proteins and healthy fats. And for many years, those that are opposed to eating animal foods have held beliefs that doing so will hurt you. Two of the top concerns are the risk of damaging your kidneys and osteoporosis. Yet, according to studies, *"It actually helps prevent damage to the kidneys,"* Dr. Sebring told me. What happens with kidney disease and failure is usually the result of high sugar and high insulin levels. Once they've been markedly damaged, then high proteins are a little tough on the kidneys. So, if you're eating a standard diet and want to prevent the damage in the first place, keep grains and carbohydrates low and increase protein.

> *"You only have three choices: fats, proteins and carbohydrates. When you cut back on your protein (proteins and fats come together) what's*

left? Carbs. And that guarantees you a continued rapid destruction of the kidneys."

As in many things, "the devil is in the details." We don't know that we have trouble with our kidneys until we've lost 80% of our kidney function. When that happens, and you've already lost 80%, it's too late; you have to cut back on protein. You might outlive that impact and your kidneys may not cause your death, but at the same time to have the health and life you deserve, you'd want to maintain an organ reserve.

"If you want to prevent yourself from getting there, the best way to do it is to eat more balanced and get plenty of protein and fat into your diet… not high carbohydrates because that is what destroys the kidneys."

Osteoporosis is admittedly a big problem in industrialized countries. What we don't hear as part of the conversation when discussing solutions is the evolutionary medicine perspective, that osteoporosis is *"absent in the archeological record prior to the institution of grains into the diet."* Time and science are showing us that many of the health problems once blaming meat as the cause, are actually caused by grains (and the many high carbohydrate processed foods made from them). Grains cause osteoporosis in two ways. One, as Dr. Sebring said, by holding magnesium in the gut, preventing it from absorbing magnesium. If you can't absorb magnesium, you can't absorb calcium. You can take calcium supplements, as is normally recommended by conventional physicians to help correct deficiency issues, but if you take them in the meal with grains you're not going to be able to absorb that calcium.

Two, grains are acidic, and by eating them our body becomes a little more acidic. The body tracks acidity very carefully and has to react if it becomes very high.

"When the ph of the blood – 7.2 or 7.4 – that's the maximum range that it is healthy. If you drop down to an acidic ph of 6.8 – 6.9, you're one sick puppy in the ICU and they're working on your hard and fast. So, that has to be carefully monitored by the body."

If there is extra acidity coming into the body, it has to get rid of that. And the way it gets rid of extra acidity is through the kidneys. As Dr. Sebring explained, the kidneys can't handle a pH lower than 5, but take someone with a urine pH of 7 (which is neutral) and give them a meal of grains, check back a little later, and they will then have a pH of 5. The kidneys are maxed out now, and they're getting rid of a whole lot of acid by buffering the urine. Guess what it buffers it with? Calcium.

So, there's two parts to this equation: input and output. The Aowin women in central Africa who get 400-500 milligrams a day of calcium in their diet don't have any osteoporosis. Why? Because the urine ph is always well above 5, so there's no need to buffer, and they don't lose calcium. And acidity problems don't just happen from grains. The second non-human food on the list is dairy. Where are the highest instances of osteoporosis in the world? Northern Europe. The same place where they have the highest dairy intake in the world, which is also very acidic.

Real Patient Results

Hearing about some of the results achieved by his patient population eating the foods they were designed to eat is impressive. Patients that have changed their cholesterol levels "beyond belief." Others that used to be diabetic are "not even close to being diabetic now," even though some are still quite a bit overweight and are still in the process of losing weight. Choosing and eating the healthiest foods—human foods—and eliminating all non-human foods, has controlled all the things "we like to measure in medicine, beautifully."

For example, one male patient, who weighs 240 pounds (he's lost 90 pounds so far), now has blood work that Dr. Sebring calls "Olympic athlete labs." He was diabetic, but no longer. He had triglycerides of 779; they are now down to 74. His HDL (good cholesterol) was a "scarily low 21", and is now up to 36. The ratio between triglycerides (fats in the body), and your HDLs (the good cholesterol), tells a doctor your insulin sensitivity; how much insulin it takes to get your sugars under control. This patient's level was 35, and now it's 2.

"This is a guy who, basically, he goes from the bed to the car, to the desk, to the car, to the couch, and to the bed. And on the weekends, you can cut out the car and the desk. But yet, he has Olympic athlete labs. That is fascinating to me. How can this be the case? It's not exercise, but it's the diet; the diet is incredibly important."

While in Wimberley, I also interviewed several of Dr. Sebring's patients who wanted to share the results they were experiencing. Because it's a small town, Steve, who owns Miss Mae's BBQ, knew Dr. Sebring casually but started seeing him as a patient because he was very concerned about his health and his future. He wasn't convinced that what he was being told to do by his conventional physician was what he should be doing. He was given multiple prescriptions: multiple blood pressure medications, beta-blockers and more. He was taking "all of these pills," and they made him feel bad. He just wasn't getting where he wanted to be.

"And so, I offered him the paleo diet, of course, and that's pretty much the first thing for anybody who comes in my clinic. They need to know that before they get out of the door, so at least they have that choice. And so he got on the diet. He did it and he did it very strictly. We would get phone calls from him, about every three of four days, about how much better he was feeling. He was checking his blood pressures at home. He's having low blood pressure now on these medications, so now he's started pulling them off... He's done so well I've not seen him in quite a while, and that's fairly typical of my paleo patients. They seem to be on auto-pilot on their health to a large degree."

A common story with patients who are following the human food diet is: they start seeing great results and start feeling better, and eating this way becomes self-perpetuating because they are doing so well. If they happen to stray from the diet, immediately they feel poorly. The negative effects of a bad diet are now easy for them to see. Dr. Sebring recalls Steve saying that when he got off the diet for a couple of days, he ended up feeling awful and started gaining a lot of weight. It took him several days to fully recover from the effects of those non-human foods once back on the proper diet. He had previously eaten a few meals that were off his diet with only slight discomfort, but those few days off were a real eye-opener for him *(See Steve's on-camera interview and other success stories at* theperfecthumandietbook.com/extras).

Collateral Healing

Another patient story is about a woman who brought her diabetic husband into the clinic for his appointment as a new patient. This couple and Dr. Sebring talked about human evolutionary nutrition, the human food and non-human food categories, and this made great sense to them. So they went home and, effectively, threw out all of their food. They went to the local health food store and stocked their cabinets, and uncharacteristically, they noticed most of the food now went into the refrigerator since fresh live foods need to be refrigerated.

She returned to the clinic two weeks later with her husband, but this time the appointment was for her. Unbeknownst to Dr. Sebring she, now in her early 60s, had fibromyalgia and chronic fatigue. She said, *"Dr. Sebring, I've had this since I was in elementary school. I had it before it was popular, before anybody knew what it was…I prayed two months ago that I would have one day without pain."* She continued the story by saying that since that first visit with her husband, it had been the finest two weeks of her life.

"I pulled the dog house into the garage the other day, scraped off all the old paint, I sanded it down, I painted it, I completed the job. I went inside and I cooked dinner for my husband. I wasn't whining and complaining about how much I hurt and how tired I was." She said, *"This is the way it's*

been for this last week, until last night." She and her husband had gone out with some friends and had Mexican food. And before she got home, all the old pain and symptoms had returned. *"I've learned an awful lot in the last two weeks."*

Another patient with depression reports that his mind is working better, his sleep is better and he's feeling happier. *"It's not a Prozac deficiency that this guy had, it's a nutritional deficiency...It's another one of those stories that you see, where finding such incredible improvement is possible, and where modern medicine wasn't getting them there."*

Dr. Sebring tells me it's these kinds of stories he finds so encouraging, and there are more stories every day from patients where these kinds of results are happening in their lives. That's why he believes we need to keep doing whatever we can to get this message out to as many people as possible. Because, like his patients, they will get it. It's too powerful once they try it.

> *"That's the virtue of this diet. It's fun. I laugh sometimes at how powerful it is, and patients look back and they laugh as well. They want to help other people and get the word out. If we can do that, if we have time to save them, then that's the question."*

The Opportunity in Correcting Course

As a viewer of the film or reader of this book, you are keenly aware that because of the radical changes to our environment and to the primary foods made available to us, we are, unfortunately, at increasingly higher risk of poor health and declining quality of life in every area, including mind and spirit. And for many, it can also mean developing severe chronic illnesses. I think you know by now that I'm an optimist, and, that with more accurate knowledge we can make the choices that will give us the health and life we deserve.

While conducting the interviews, I asked some of the scientists and researchers if it was too late for us. Our species. Had we gone over the edge of the waterfall and there was just no way to recover?

Dr. Sebring, as usual, was straightforward.

"I don't know the answer to that. I have to be an optimist here, and I have to try. If you have eight doors to open and only one will get you there, and if you don't open any, it's over. You'd better open one door at least. I'm trying to get the word out. And we're growing here, in the small town of Wimberley, and now (with the film) we have the opportunity here to bring this to the world. I have to be optimistic about it. Like I said, I'm a romanticist and I think we'll survive."

As our conversation was winding down, we talked a bit about environmental factors that can harm us. We've created chemicals that never before existed on the earth. Pollutants and plastics can cause disease. Heavy metals are another. Huge amounts of stress are a fourth one. But the number one thing you can do something about the most easily, as an individual, is the diet. And that gives you the strength to continue attacking the others.

"The body can detoxify a lot of those chemicals and heavy metals much more efficiently if you're eating human foods. If you give the cells the nutrition they need, then they can perform the functions they were designed to perform. And if you're not giving them the nutrition they need, if you're giving them toxins from the non-human foods, you don't have a chance. You're guaranteed to lose, and we're seeing it. Everybody hurts, everybody's overweight and they don't know what to do about it. So, here's our opportunity; we're hanging on by our fingertips."

Hunt: "So, take the opportunity."

Dr. Sebring: *"Please. Try it. Like I said, the diet self-perpetuates and people feel better than they've ever felt. Things go away that they didn't even know were a problem. A guy comes in today and says, the ringing in my ears is gone, and the grinding in my neck is gone. I only did this diet in support of my wife, who is trying to lose weight, but I feel good. I sleep like a baby."*
"And I hear these stories all day long."

Part Three
THE "HOW TO"

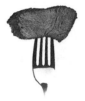

THE PERFECT HUMAN DIET™
THE NEXT WAVE IN DIET & HEALTH

Chapter 10

"No idea is so complex that it can't be explained simply"
—**Albert Einstein**

N ow that you come this far it should be pretty clear that *The Perfect Human Diet* companion books purpose is to help you put these species specific, optimal method of eating into practice in a simple, straightforward way. This method of eating is not the kind of prescriptive diet program you may be most familiar with, using instead, easy, solution driven distinctions in order to maximize your success in reaching your optimal health and wellness goals. This intentional approach, defining foods into our two lists, reinforces unconscious competence so you won't have to struggle with choosing what food to eat, no matter what circumstances you find yourself in.

Viewers have written me on numerous occasions since the film premiered, sharing their successes in transforming their health and well-being after watching the film. Why did watching a movie make the difference for them? Because they could finally see and understand the full story of human nutrition. The conclusions and food recommendations made perfect sense to them, and were very easy for them to start doing. My hope is that this "how-to" companion to the film will do the same for you too with the added advantage of some detail, directions and recipes which couldn't be provided in the film. I also hope that you're excited about launching the next chapter of your personal human nutrition story.

Let's get started.

The Perfect Human Diet™ "How-To" Overview

1. Eat whole and fresh foods from the PHD[49] Human Food list.
2. Eat primarily animal foods and fats.
3. Eat non-starchy veggies as desired with meals.
4. Eat low-sugar fruits, fresh nuts and seeds (in moderation).
5. Eat whenever you're hungry.
6. Forget calorie counting. Let your hunger, which is in sync with your activity level, be your guide on how much to eat.
7. Drink plenty of pure water (coffee and tea ok).

*Of course, be as active as you can, and get a good night's sleep.

In addition, most people will benefit by including these three supplements daily: Omega 3s from fish oil, Acidophilus (a probiotic) and a quality multi-vitamin (for suggested brands see Resources or www.theperfecthumandietbook.com/extras).

The Basics: *Simplicity Is Your Best Friend*

The meal guide below is designed to comfortably apply to the widest range of reader's world-wide. That said, there is a "*Good, Better, Best*"

---

49   PHD: Acronym for "Perfect Human Diet"

hierarchy for meats, poultry and eggs available in the U.S. Those U.S. distinctions are in the chapter on shopping.

#1 Each meal should start with a major source of animal protein. Be sure to eat it to your satisfaction. For example:
- Beef, lamb, pork, veal, game, organ meats, rabbit.
- All fish and seafood.
- Poultry: chicken, duck, quail, pheasant, squab.
- Eggs of all kinds (The variety I saw in Europe is astounding.)

Reporter's notes:

You can now easily find organic and grass-fed meats and poultry in a growing number of traditional grocery stores, or online if you plan ahead.

#2 You can add any variety or quantity of non-starchy vegetables at any meal, especially above the ground leafy vegetables.
- Fresh and uncooked in salads.
- Organic if possible, avoiding the "Dirty Dozen™"[50] (see shopping tips).
- Lightly steamed, or gently stir fried in a heat appropriate human food oil
- In soups made with an animal based stock (good ones can be had in the freezer section of any supermarkets, or online).
- Homemade stocks from the bones of chicken, beef, lamb or fish are nice to use in your cooking when you can.
- Meat stocks are a great base for sauces too.

Reporter's notes:

Corn, which is often thought of as an above the ground vegetable in our country, is actually a grain - part of the Non-Human food list.

---

50   Source: Environmental Working Group, www.ewg.org

#3 Eat only Human Food Fats and Oils

- Animal fats that naturally occur in organic grass fed and pastured meats and poultry, or wild seafood and game.
- Rendered animal fats from organic pastured grass-fed such as tallow and lard.
- Some plant oils such as expeller pressed extra-virgin olive oil (it'll say this on the label), sesame oil, and virgin cold-pressed tropical oils e.g. coconut oil and palm oil.
- Butter and ghee from grass-fed animals is OK.

#4 Eat fresh raw nuts, seeds and nut butters

- Moderate amounts.
- Not "peanuts or peanut butter" as they are not really nuts they're legumes - a non-human food.

#5 Eat a variety of low sugar fresh fruits and berries

- Preferably organic
- In small amounts.
- As a simple dessert.
- Between meals with a few fresh nuts.

Reporter's notes:

If you have known allergies, or unexpected allergic reactions to any of these foods, or other unlisted foods, follow your health provider's instructions to avoid or eliminate as necessary.

Next up, shopping tips.

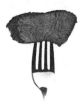

SHOPPING TIPS

Chapter 11

Most people still shop in regular supermarkets, so when it comes to meats, fish and poultry it's good to know there IS a hierarchy of preferred sources - a "good, better and best" - version of that particular food. Luckily the full range of these preferred animal foods are becoming more widely available.

Animal Foods and Seafoods: *Good, Better, Best*
1. **Best:** Comes from animals that are pasture raised, eating the foods they were designed to eat. This also includes wild game of all kinds and fresh wild-caught or wild harvested seafoods.
2. **Better:** Organically raised meats, organic free-range poultry.
3. **Good:** "Naturally" raised meats or poultry.

Plant Foods: *Fruits and Vegetables*
When it comes to knowing which commercially grown fruits and vegetables are better to buy organic, and avoiding the ones that retain

the most pesticides, plant foods that make the Human Food list have a hierarchy as well, what I simply call the "Best" and "Worst" for you. The most well-known and respected resource for pesticide residue on commercial fruits and vegetables is the Environmental Working Group Organization (EWG) who publishes the popular "Dirty Dozen™" and "Clean Fifteen™" lists. Nicely enough they gave me permission to reprint their lists here. You will also find their handy food shoppers guide graphics in the Resources section so you can clip it out to take along while food shopping.

Plant Foods: *The Worst for You*

The following commercially grown fruits and vegetables have the highest pesticide load it's always best to buy them organically grown. (Items marked with * are not on the PHD Human Food list).

Apples
Celery
Cherry tomatoes
Cucumbers
Grapes
Nectarines (imported)
Peaches
Snap peas* (imported)
Spinach
Strawberries
Sweet bell peppers
Potatoes*

EWG has developed a "Plus +" category now too. These are listed "highly toxic" and of special concern when it comes to your health and wellness:

- Hot peppers
- Kale/Collards

Plant Foods: *The Best for You*

These "Clean Fifteen™" foods had the lowest amount of pesticides leaving residue. These are conventionally grown crops that are OK to consume from the standpoint of the least pesticide contamination. Of course, organic is preferred whenever possible.

Asparagus
Avocados
Cabbage
Cantaloupe
Cauliflower
Eggplant
Grapefruit
Kiwi
Mangoes
Onions
Papayas
Pineapples
Sweet Corn*
Sweet Peas* (frozen)
Sweet Potatoes*

Copyright © Environmental Working Group, www.ewg.org. Reprinted with permission.

Imported fruits and vegetables, unfortunately, may still contain herbicides and pesticides that have been banned in the United States. The lesson here of course is, even with fruits and vegetables, look at the labels to see its country of origin. You might also double check with the manager of the supermarket you shop in. I mention this because managers at Trader Joe's tell me their buyers have made site visits, at least in Mexico, to verify organic sources. Also some major health food store chains say they too verify their sources. It can't hurt to ask your stores management though, especially given the ongoing changes in worldwide food distribution systems. Clearly, it's great if and when you can get these preferred sources of animal foods and plant foods.

You'd be hard-pressed to find someone who doesn't think that they taste better too.

Availability

The really great news is that major superstore chains like Wal-Mart, Costco, Ralph's, Kroger's and others are rapidly incorporating organic fresh and organic frozen foods into their stores. They are also offering organic foods at much lower prices than found in the biggest U.S. health food store chain. With animal foods in particular, I've found these new offerings often include an unexpected range of choices.

For example in my local Ralph's supermarket they now carry Organic grass-fed[51] beef, organic chicken,[52] "naturally raised" selections, and of course the standard USDA grades of meats and poultry. They also often feature wild caught seafoods and fish. A new addition to many supermarket egg departments worth checking out is a new pasture raised egg brand that originated in the UK called "Happy Eggs."[53] But make no mistake, having this new variety of foods available is a consumer driven movement, one that, with your participation, is growing stronger every day. So, if for some reason your local supermarket chain hasn't climbed on board the organic and grass-fed movement yet, it can't hurt to give a friendly request to the stores manager.

Should you have access to a more specialized fresh foods supermarket, or a local Farmer's Market that has a wider variety of fresh seasonal fruits and vegetables, certainly take advantage of that whenever you can. If you haven't explored Farmers Markets they can be quite an adventure and pretty remarkable. Some include vendors that bring in locally sourced organic and grass-fed meats of all kinds, wild-caught seafoods and the eggs and meat from pastured raised poultry that has scratched around in their

---

51 Most often means they were raised through most of their life on organic grass, but the government does allow producers to use other organic feed for a short time just before processing.* "Grass finished" is a newer labeling distinction allowing consumers who want only grass fed meats to be sure they are purchasing it.

52 Organic feed can still include corn and soy.

53 More info see thehappyeggco.com

own yard and nicely enough, seen sunlight. The bottom line here is, any time we can expand the varieties of Human Foods we eat, we get a wider range of nutrients to support our health and well-being.

Don't Throw out the Baby

It's worth acknowledging that in industrialized countries commercially raised fresh and frozen foods are still what dominate the available food landscape. If you can't get the best sources of the PHD Human Foods where you live, when you're out and about or traveling, you can certainly eat commercially raised meat and plant foods from the Human Foods list. In fact it's pretty easy to optimize the health benefits of commercial foods and your overall diet while minimizing the potential of any negative effects to your health. The three top suggestions would be, 1) trim the excess fat off of commercially raised meats, 2) eat more of the best fats from the human food list, and 3) take the top three supplements Dr. Sebring recommends. A few suggested brands are in the Resources section or online at *www.theperfecthumandietbook.com/extras*.

Read the Labels (yes, again)

It's true that needing to read the labels on anything you might buy prepackaged virtually every time you go shopping can be a bit of a hassle. As it turns out, even simple straightforward kitchen basics aren't safe from their ingredients shifting due to supply chain and manufacturing issues that arise. A quick example that comes to mind is jarred organic Dijon mustard from a nationally known, upscale health food store chain. In this particular case, apple cider vinegar became just vinegar, without any source information. It caught my eye only because I had made a real effort to seek out the healthiest version I could find, like I do now for all foods. Considering it has such a short list of ingredients, this was unexpected. This change of ingredients over time held true for other items I occasionally purchased pre-made as well, such as organic chicken and vegetable broth.

"Low-Fat Guacamole" (a cautionary tale)

But what finally made me a hard-core label reader was this. You may find it as hard to believe as I did when I first discovered it. Ever heard of "low-fat guacamole?" [54] Neither had I, until I picked up an in-house made container of guacamole from the cold deli case of a nationally known, upscale health food store chain. In large letters at the top of the label was "Low-fat Guacamole" followed by all the small print that, at first glance, looked like a pretty standard guacamole recipe, all the things you'd expect. But, as it turned out, the method they used to make it "low-fat" was by adding *sugar*. Growing up in California eating lots of guacamole I had never heard of a recipe that added sugar, but doing so certainly achieved the desired lower-fat outcome. It changed the macronutrient ratios driving down the percentage of fat in the guacamole. All I can say after that is, seems like a good idea to keep reading labels.

Reporter's Notes: "Good, Better, Best"

While you will certainly want to be mindful about eating only the very best foods if you're healing from, or living with, a chronic medical condition (as I am), even without supplementation you'll be way ahead of the game by eating only the Human Foods listed in the next chapter.[55]

If you want to keep updated on any changes or additions to our PHD Human Food and Non-Human food lists vetted by our first-person scientific and medical sources (along with new film projects, production news and resources) please see my blog at CJHuntReports.com. The food lists will also be updated in www.theperfecthumandietbook.com/extras.

---

54 I also found a commercial brand of guacamole in California doing the same thing, at the same nationally known store.

55 Of course always seek out the council of a knowledgeable evolutionary health practitioner who can help you design the best course of action for your personal circumstances.

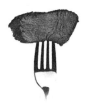

HUMAN FOOD & NON-HUMAN FOOD

Chapter 12

"For my patients sake, and in some ways for myself, I sort of break food into two categories: human food, and non-human food. And the human foods would be: the lean meats, turkey, fish, chicken... preferably from an animal that was eating what it was designed to eat... fruits, nuts and vegetables.

The non-human food would be: the grains, which is probably the worst problem that we have; dairy, after two years old; we're not designed for dairy after two years old, certainly not from another animal; and beans and potatoes.

And so, those are the simple categories that I put them in... and people understand that, I understand that, and it helps me to make choices."

—Dr. Lane Sebring to C.J. Hunt in his documentary, *The Perfect Human Diet*

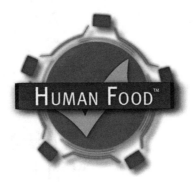

#1 Animal Proteins (whole cuts are best)

Bear
Beef
Bison
Chicken
Duck
Free range eggs
Elk
Wild caught fish
Goat
Goose
Lamb
Organ meats
Ostrich
Pork
Rabbit
Shellfish
Turkey
Venison

Reporter's Notes: "Lean Meats"

To put this in context, while shooting the film Dr. Sebring and I were discussing commercially raised meats available to most people. In these instances, choosing lean cuts or trimming off excess fat is a good idea.

Then just be sure to eat some of the healthy human fats with that meal. If you get pastured, grass fed meat, that fat is very good for you, and the "lean meats" reference doesn't apply.

#2 VEGETABLES (all preferably Organic)

Acorn squash

Artichokes

Arugula

Asparagus

Avocado (technically a fruit)

Bamboo shoots

Beet greens

Beets

Bok Choy

Broccoli

Broccoli Rabi

Brussels sprouts

Butternut squash

Cabbage

Carrots

Cauliflower

Celery

Chard

Collard greens

Cucumber

Daikon radish

Delicata squash

Eggplant

Endive

Escarole

Fennel

Jicama

Kale

Kohlrabi
Leek
Lettuce
Mushroom
Mustard greens
Pickles
Pumpkin
Radicchio
Radishes
Rhubarb
Rutabaga
Scallions
Shallots
Spaghetti squash
Spinach
Summer squash
Sweet/hot peppers
Tomato
Turnip greens
Turnips
Watercress
Zucchini

#3 FATS & OILS (all preferably Organic)

Avocado oil, extra virgin
Coconut oil, extra virgin and virgin
Olive oil, extra virgin first press
Palm oil
Macadamia oil
Sesame oil
Tallow, Grass-fed Beef
Walnut oil

Reporter's Notes: Fats and Dairy

Dr. Sebring's practice has proven two exceptions that help his patient's dietary changes easier to incorporate.

Butter: from Grass-fed cows.* Most people will not have any negative health ramifications. *Not a Human Food, but OK.

Ghee: clarified from grass-fed source butter. The harmful milk proteins are separated out, leaving only the fat.

#4 NUTS/SEEDS (all preferably Organic)

Almonds
Brazil nuts
Chestnuts
Chia
Coconut
Flax seeds
Macadamia
Pecans
Pine nuts
Pistachio
Pumpkin seeds
Sesame seeds
Sunflower seeds
Walnuts

#5 FRUIT (all preferably Organic)

Apples
Apricots
Asian pear
Banana
Blackberries
Blueberries
Boysenberries
Cantaloupe

Cherries
Clementine
Cranberries
Currents
Dates
Figs
Grapefruit
Grapes
Honeydew
Melon
Kiwi
Kumquats
Lemon
Lime
Mango
Medjool Date
Nectarine
Orange
Papaya
Passion fruit
Peach
Pear
Persimmon
Pineapple
Plantain
Plums
Pomegranate
Quince

Reporter's Notes:

With fruits, preferentially *eat low sugar varieties*. I've found having a little bit of low-sugar fruit as a dessert right after a meal makes it easy not to overindulge.

HERBS/SPICES (all preferably Organic)

Basil
Chili powder
Chives
Cilantro
Cinnamon
Cloves
Cumin
Garlic
Ginger
Honey
Maple syrup (*very small amounts)
Marjoram
Mint
Molasses (*very small amounts)
Mustard
Nutmeg
Oregano
Paprika
Parsley
Pepper
Rosemary
Saffron
Sage
Seaweed
Thyme
Turmeric
Vanilla

Reporter's Notes:

Unless you know the source, use single spices only and mix your own combinations. Commercially available spice combinations can hide toxic ingredients not listed on the label.

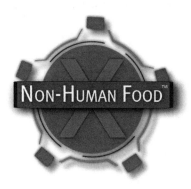

"The non-human food would be: the grains, which is probably the worst problem that we have; dairy, after two years old; we're not designed for dairy after two years old, certainly not from another animal; beans and potatoes."

—Dr. Lane Sebring to C.J. Hunt
in his documentary *The Perfect Human Diet*

To keep it simple, the doctor has whittled it down to these four food groups.

#1 GRAINS
Don't eat anything made from grain. Common grains include: wheat, buckwheat, millet, oatmeal or oats, quinoa, amaranth, rice, barley and rye. Common products include bread, pasta, baked goods (like cookies, cakes and crackers), cereals, doughnuts and grain flours.

#2 DAIRY
Milk, cheese and yogurt. Products made from dairy, such as sour cream, cream cheese, reduced fat milks, ice cream.

Reporter's Notes:

Dr. Sebring's one exception is butter from organic grass-fed cows. You can of course replace butter with other healthy human food fats such as coconut oil.

#3 BEANS(legumes)

All kinds. No exceptions. For example: soy beans, green beans, peas, chickpeas, garbanzo beans, kidney beans, lima beans, black beans, white beans, navy beans, pinto beans. Products made from beans, for example: processed soy products like tofu, soy milk, veggie burgers, soy cheese, soy yogurt.

#4 Potatoes (aka tubers)

All kinds. No exceptions (including sweet potatoes and yams). There are many varieties, but those all fit into just a few categories, such as: russet potatoes, yellow potatoes (aka Yukon), white potatoes, red potatoes and blue-purple potatoes. Products made from potatoes such as chips, French fries, dehydrated mashed potatoes, potato flour.

Reporter's Notes:

As Dr. Sebring told me during our supermarket tour, almost everything in a modern food store is a Non-Human food and isn't good for us.

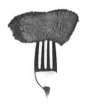

THE HUMAN FOOD KITCHEN

Chapter 13

Set Yourself up to Win

Like any significant change in habits, at least in the food department, setting yourself up to be successful can be done in a few easy steps. As they used to say when I was a kid, "out with the old, and in with the new!"

1. Make room in the kitchen and cupboards for a few days worth of fresh, healthy, Human Foods so the foods that will bring you optimal health are handy when you're hungry.
2. Take the Non-Human food out of your cupboards and refrigerator and dispose of it.

If you feel a bit uncomfortable with just tossing it all out, and they are unopened or in good enough shape, a local church that has a food program might like them. Of course, many communities also have "Meals on Wheels" nonprofit organizations to help feed folks who are too sick or elderly for many simple tasks such as shopping and cooking, and the might be grateful for your contribution.

Suggested Basic Kitchen Items

Raw nuts and seeds (best to keep in your freezer), e.g., Almond, Walnuts, Pecans, Brazil nuts, Pine nuts, Pumpkin seeds, Sunflower seeds.

Coconut flakes, Organic, unsweetened (or shredded Coconuts).

Almond butter, Organic, creamy or crunchy (For the adventurous, sunflower butter and macadamia butter are easy to find).

In addition to your favorite herbs and spices, this list includes the needed ingredients for the "Perfect Human Comfort Food Recipes" in the next chapter. Always get them organic where possible.

Arrowroot.
Baking soda.
Bay Leaf.
Black pepper.
Cinnamon.
Nutmeg.
Cloves.
Ground mace.
Dark chili powder.
Dried oregano.
Onion powder.
Poppy seeds.
Sesame seeds.
Flax seeds.
Caraway seeds.
Onion Flakes.
Sea salt.
Vanilla extract.
Organic Chicken stock.
Sun dried tomatoes.

Organic Dijon mustard.

Organic canned tomatoes.

Tomato paste.

Olives.

Almond Flour *(called Almond Meal at Trader Joe's).*

Blanched Almond Flour.

Coconut flour.

Organic grass-fed butter.

Yacon syrup *(for Price-Pottenger Nutrition Foundations Pumpkin Bread).*

Oils: Extra virgin olive oil. Extra virgin or virgin coconut oil. Walnut oil. If possible keep all of your liquid oil soils refrigerated. This helps minimize oxidation and maintain flavor.

*The exception to refrigeration is coconut oil which can be used for cooking or, like grass-fed butter, eating.

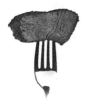

PERFECT HUMAN
COMFORT FOOD RECIPES

Chapter 14

P eople have written me with many types of questions after watching the film, but one of the easiest to answer is how to best emulate the tastes and textures of comfort foods they grew up with. Partly because they love those foods, and also because they have failed in the past with other diets because it wasn't possible to make great tasting and satisfying comfort foods from the foods allowed on those diets.

The beauty of *The Perfect Human Diet* is that you don't have to give up having comfort foods and wonderful meals to create the health and life you deserve. Here are some great tasting recipes using PHD Human Foods that are the creation of my good friend and Hunt Thompson Media Managing Partner, George Thompson. George was raised in an Italian household in Connecticut, and luckily his culinary skills were learned while observing his Italian mother and grandmother. Both of these women were real sticklers for fresh homemade food, made from scratch, and George started absorbing their family secrets while doing his elementary school homework at the kitchen table.

Years later, George started doing a lot of cooking on his own and, thanks to a little extra direction from his mom, mastered the home made make it from scratch skills. A skill set much appreciated by his friends and dinner guests over the years (including me). I hope you enjoy them too.

SMALL BITES
Seeded Almond Flatbread
Baked Mini Meat Balls
Banana Walnut Muffins
Pepper and Eggs

SOUPS AND SALADS
Nothing but a Green Salad
Summer Tomato Salad
A New Face for Tuna Salad
Fish Chowder
Quick Homemade Tomato Soup

MAIN DISHES
Thursday Night was Pasta Night
Pasta Substitutes
Italian Stewed Stuffed Pork Chops
Pot Roast/Beef Stew (but forget the potatoes)
Chili (no beans)
The Sunday Roast - Roast Pork with Apple Sauce
The Sunday Roast II - Roast Chicken with Whipped Cauliflower
A Holiday Meal Dressing for your Bird

NEXT DAY LEFTOVERS
Next Day Shepherd's Pie
Chili Dog
Egg Crepes Sweet or Savory (who needs pancakes)
Cauliflower Patties
Next Day Classic Chicken Soup

DESSERTS
All American Apple Pie (almost)
Pumpkin Bread

Seeded Almond Flatbread

I fondly remember the Everything Bagel I used to get on the run in NYC years ago, sometimes toasted with cream cheese. This is a great substitute that captures the taste and texture of the seeded toasted bagel and goes with appetizers, soups or main courses alike. My favorite way of eating them is with a pat of Kerry Gold butter with thin slices of radishes on top.

1 cup almond flour
½ tsp sea salt
¼ tsp onion powder
1 large egg white
½ tsp raw flax seeds
½ tsp sesame seeds
½ tsp poppy seeds
½ tsp onion flakes

Combine almond flour, salt & onion powder in medium mixing bowl.

Add one egg white (I keep the extra yolk to add to the breakfast scramble)…Mix well with a large spoon or spatula until a smooth texture is achieved…Form into a disc and place on parchment paper.

Place plastic wrap on top and roll out (I use a French rolling pin as it gives better control when rolling out the dough – this recipe will easily fill a 14"x12" cookie sheet).

Remove the plastic wrap, sprinkle the seeds and onion flakes on top, place plastic wrap back on and gently roll the seeds into the dough, remove plastic wrap again and score the dough to the desired shapes or bake whole and break apart after it is cooked for an artisan look.

Bake for 10-12 minutes in a 340 degree preheated oven.

They should be lightly browned, but not too dark, as they will burn quickly.

Cool for about 2 minutes, remove the parchment paper and snap apart.

Store in a sealed container to maintain the crisp!

Baked Mini Meat Balls

This is a great appetizer, snack or fun lunch for kids and adults alike. They taste more like hamburgers since we add no breadcrumbs they are great to eat with different dipping sauces or relishes.

1 lb ground beef or buffalo (85/15 is perfect)
1/8 tsp onion powder
1/8 tsp garlic powder
1 tsp dried oregano
2 tbsp olive oil
Salt and black pepper to taste

Form meat into very small one-bite balls no bigger than 1 inch in diameter.

Bake on a cookie sheet in a 400 degree oven for about 12 minutes, turning once at the six minute mark.

Remove to a mixing bowl drizzle in olive oil, add spices, toss and serve.

Banana Walnut Muffins
(2 bites and sugar free)

I spent many summers with my sister at her lake house. She used to make banana nut bread, so this is my comfort food I got from her.

I think bananas and walnuts were a marriage made in heaven. Walk into any coffee shop and you will see a huge selection of baked goods, but when did those muffins start looking like they are some science experiment growing to unnatural sizes? These muffins are great for breakfast or afternoon snack with a cup of tea or coffee. No need for any added sugar if the banana is extra ripe it should satisfy your sweet cravings.

1 large very ripe banana
1 cup blanched almond flour
1 large egg
1 tbsp butter
¼ tsp salt
½ tsp baking soda
1/8 tsp vanilla extract
1/3 cup chopped walnuts

Melt the butter.

Mash the banana, add the melted butter, egg and vanilla extract and blend well.

Add all the remaining dry ingredients and continue to mix until filly incorporated.

Add the walnuts in my hand with a spatula.

Spoon batter into the 12 mini-muffin wells that have been slightly pregreased with butter.

Bake at 325 degrees for about 17-20 minutes.

Let cool in the muffin tin for a few minutes, remove and let cool for at least another 15 minutes on rack. (I have found the flavor to be more intense when the muffins are cooled down or even kept until the next day).

Pepper and Eggs

I loved this for breakfast, lunch or dinner when I was a kid. But my mother used to fry the peppers in olive oil and that was messy and took too much time. So roasting the red peppers are better and easier... and taste just as good.

> 2 red bell peppers
> 3 tbsp olive oil
> 4 eggs beaten
> Salt and black pepper to taste

Roast two red sweet bell peppers on a cookie sheet in a toaster oven on 475 degrees for about 30 - 35 minutes.

Remove and immediately wrap in aluminum foil and let sit for another 30 minutes. After 30 minutes the skins will easily peel off.

Slit the pepper in half and scoop out the seeds and core.

Cut into strips and reserve with two tablespoons of olive oil (You can prepare the peppers a day in advance, as they will keep in the refrigerator, if you don't eat them first).

Heat pan to medium high heat, add one Tbsp of olive oil.

Add your prepared red peppers and heat them for a minute before pouring in the 4 beaten eggs.

Keep mixing the two together as the eggs cook. (You will never want plain scrambled eggs again).

Nothing but a Green Salad

Growing up we always ate a green salad at the end of the meal (tomatoes were never added and in fact we only ate tomatoes in their own salad and only in the summer with tomatoes fresh off the vine from my grandfather's garden). The salad was always the same: iceberg lettuce, scallions and cucumbers in an olive oil and apple cider vinegar dressing. Don't resort to bottled salad dressing, fresh is always better (and opening up two bottles is just as easy as one). Our salad is slightly different, but has the same spirit of my families only green salad.

1 small head of organic iceberg lettuce (yes organic
does make a big difference here in the texture)
1 small head of green butter lettuce
2-3 scallions
1 small peeled cucumber
2-3 white radishes

Wash and dry very well all the greens, residual water will ruin your dressing.

Tear apart the lettuce leaves, cut the scallion into ½ inch pieces, and slice the cucumber and radishes thinly.

Salt and pepper, add about ¼ cup good extra virgin 1st press olive oil and 2 Tbsp of the vinegar.

Toss until greens are coated; adjust seasoning and oil/vinegar for taste.

Summer Tomato Salad

So now that I told you we never added tomatoes to our green salad, I guess you'd like to know how we ate tomatoes. Very simply, and only in the summertime when they were vine ripened. The Italians seem to love food that has the colors of their flag, so the red of the tomato, the green of the pepper and oregano and the white was the piece of bread that usually accompanied the salad. But skip the bread, as this is just as good without it.

1 large ripe tomato, cut into bite sized pieces
½ tsp dried oregano
2-3 tbsp olive oil
Salt to taste
1 Green Cayenne Hot Pepper cut into small pieces (optional)

In a medium bowl mix all ingredients together and let sit at room temperature for about 5 minutes to let the tomatoes release their juice and mix with the oil. (Never use a cold tomato; the cold kills the taste in my opinion).

Serve and enjoy.

A New Face For Tuna Salad

Who doesn't remember the old tuna salad standby, but with the mayonnaises today made with unhealthy oils and no time to make your own healthy mayo, this is a quick and easy twist to an old favorite. It makes a great lunch or dinner entrée salad.

Baby arugula, prewashed
1 small red onion, sliced
2 cans of tuna, drained of their liquid
2 celery stalks, chopped
4 tbs Olive oil
2 tbs Apple cider vinegar
Juice of ½ lemon
½ teas dill
Salt and black pepper to taste

Combine the arugula, red onion, celery and tuna in a large salad bowl.

Salt and pepper the dry salad mixture.

Mix the oil, vinegar, lemon and dill in a cup and pour over the salad.

Toss and serve with our flatbread as a quick, easy and satisfying meal.

Fish Chowder

Whether you grew up in New England like me or not, fish chowders or gumbos are so much a part of comfort food lists. This one uses arrowroot instead of flour and skips the potatoes, but is still hearty and a perfect substitute.

2 – 3 cups fish stock (depending on how much broth you like)
1 lb of Cod pieces
1 lb of Mahi-Mahi cut into bite-size pieces
3 - 4 stalks of celery and their leaves cut into 1-inch pieces
1 large onion chopped
1 clove garlic minced
6 - 8 large okra cut into 1-inch pieces
2 tbsp butter
2 tsp arrowroot
¼ cup fresh chopped parsley
Salt and white pepper to taste

Melt butter in your stock-pot, add the arrowroot and brown slightly on a medium heat.

Add the okra, garlic, celery stalk pieces (not the leaves) and onions and cook for 2 minutes.

Add in the fish stock and the fish, celery leaves, parsley, salt and pepper.

Let simmer for 1 hour to 90 minutes.

The cod pieces should break and along with the okra up to help give the soup a thickness.

I like to cool the soup down and refrigerate and reheat it the next day after all the flavors have had time to meld together.

Quick Homemade Tomato Soup

If you grew up in the 1950's or 1960's like me, Tomato Soup was iconic and remains a comfort food, reminding me of coming in from the snow or rain, warming up and mom. This version, not as quick as opening up a can, is a bit more adult with the added fresh shallots and basil. Eat it with our flatbread recipe and some cold meat and it's the perfect substitute for the soup and sandwich combo. This soup will keep in the refrigerator for several days afterwards so feel free to double the batch.

28oz can of peeled ground organic tomatoes
8oz organic chicken stock
2 chopped shallots
2 tbsp chopped fresh basil
2 tbsp olive oil
Salt and black pepper to taste

Heat olive oil in a 2-quart saucepan.

Add the shallots and cook over a medium heat for about 5-10 minutes.

Add the tomatoes, stock, basil and salt and black pepper.

Stir, cover and let simmer for about 20 minutes.

Using an emersion wand, blend the tomatoes in. If you like a chucky soup then blend only slightly.

Stir and let it cook for 5 more minutes.

Main Dishes

Thursday Night was Pasta Night

Growing up in an Italian household, we had pasta every Thursday night, so how could I give it up. Well I don't, I now understand the pasta was the least significant part of the meal, it was the rich tomato sauce with three meats that cooked all day in the sauce that made it memorable and my ultimate comfort food.

Classic Red Sauce

1 Green bell pepper
1 Red bell pepper
2 cloves of garlic
1 large onion or 2 medium onions
1 small can of tomato paste
4 large cans of whole tomatoes
¼ cup chopped flat leaf parsley
1 tsp dried oregano
Olive oil
Salt & black pepper to taste

Skin and cut the bell peppers into a small dice, small dice onion, peel the garlic clove.

Heat pan with olive oil, sweat the peppers with the onion for about 10 minutes, push to side of pan, add a bit more olive oil if needed, then add in the tomato paste and whole garlic cloves.

Soften the garlic until it can be easily crushed with the back end of a fork. Brown the paste slowly until it turns a dark red brown.

Add the chopped parsley and incorporate the pepper and onions into the paste, garlic and parsley.

Meanwhile, crush the whole tomatoes through a strainer to remove any seeds (seeds will make the sauce bitter (this way there is no need to add sugar as my grandmother used to say, its takes a little more effort but its worth it).

Bring the crushed tomatoes to a low simmer.

Add the paste mixture to the tomatoes.

Deglaze the paste pan to get any remaining bits out and add to the saucepot.

Let simmer on low for a minimum of 3 hours. Stir occasionally and add water of it gets too thick (although I don't think it can ever be too thick.)

Meats to add to the Classic Red Sauce

Adding meat to your sauce is very important as the meat will flavor the sauce and the sauce will tenderize and flavor the meat. I've eliminated meatballs from this recipe, although my grandmother made the best meatballs, she used breadcrumbs in the mixture. Instead, I brown chopped sirloin in olive oil and just add the crumbled meat to the sauce.

1 rack of baby back pork ribs
1 piece of hot Italian sausage
1 piece of mild Italian sausage
1 lb chopped beef sirloin

Preheat the oven to 350 degrees, cut your pork ribs into 3 rib pieces, and your hot and mild Italian sausage into 1 inch pieces.

Bake them for about 45 minutes to get the excess fat out of the meats, and then add them to sauce.

When the sauce is finished cooking, remove the pork ribs and sausages so that everyone can get a piece of each.

Pasta Substitutes

With these two pasta substitutes, Thursday nights can always be pasta night or invite your friends over and celebrate Abbondonza!

1) Roasted Eggplant Lasagna

Slice the eggplant in thin slices, brush with olive oil and roast in the oven at 350 degrees until tender.

Layer the slices in a lasagna pan with the meat sauce, bake in a 325 degree oven for about 1 hour. Serve with sausage and ribs on the side. You wont miss the pasta, I promise you!

2) Zucchetti (blanched spiraled zucchini)

Buy a spiral vegetable slicer; it is well worth the $40. This kitchen tool easily makes thin pasta-like spirals out of zucchini in seconds. What's wonderful about Zucchetti is the neutral flavor of the zucchini that allows the taste of our Classic Red sauce come front and center, unlike what I've experienced with Spaghetti Squash.

Allow 1 to 1½ zucchini per person.

Blanch spirals in boiling water for about 90 seconds to 2 minutes.

Drain and toss with our classic red sauce.

Italian Stewed Stuffed Pork Chops

When I'm craving that tomato sauce and meat combination but don't have the time to make my grandmother's red sauce, I find this meal is a great substitute. Easy to make and practically cooks itself.

4 Boneless thick pork chops
Salt and black pepper to taste
1 medium onion chopped
1 clove minced garlic
2 tbsp olive oil
4 Roma tomatoes chopped
8 Sundried tomatoes
8 Fresh basil leaves

Slice a pocket in the pork chops and stuff two basil leaves and 2 sundried tomatoes inside each chop.

Salt and pepper the chops and brown in the olive oil.

Add the onions, garlic and the tomatoes on top and around the chops.

Add just a ¼ cup of red wine or water.

Cover and let simmer for 90 minutes to 2 hours.

Pot Roast/Beef Stew
(but forget the potatoes)

My mom used to make the best beef stew and pot roast the meat would fall apart in your mouth and the rich gravy was then sopped up with a piece of crusty Italian bread. This version eliminates the potatoes and flour my mom used to thicken the liquid, but the meat is as tender and the broth is a wonderful beef onion flavor. I add the leeks to this for onion variety and color. So eat the meat and vegetable with a folk, but have a soupspoon on hand afterwards for the broth. This recipe works for stew meat, or a roast.

2lbs beef stew meat or one 3 lb pot roast
1 large onion cut into bit size pieces
1 large leek sliced into 1-inch pieces
4 carrots cut into 1-inch pieces
1 clove garlic chopped
¼ cup chopped flat leaf parsley
1 bay leaf
Butter for cooking
Salt
Black pepper

Pat meat dry. In an enamel cast iron pot melt 1tbsp butter. Brown the meat, and then remove. Add 1 more tbsp butter and sweat the leek and onion.

Add back the meat. Add the carrots, parsley, salt and pepper to taste and the bay leaf.

Add 2 cups water, cover and simmer for 2 to 3 hours.

Chili (no beans)

Cold autumn nights, a bowl of chili and a green salad were a Saturday night treat eaten on the TV tray in the living room - the only night of the week I was allowed to eat that way.

2 lbs of ground sirloin (90/10)
5 to 6 Roma tomatoes chopped
1 large onion
2 tbsp olive oil
1 tsp tomato paste
1 tsp of mustard
1-2 tbsp of dark chili power
½ tsp of dried oregano
2 tbsp chopped parsley
½ tsp dried dill
Salt and pepper to taste

Heat olive oil in a chili pot, sweat the onions on medium for about 5 min, push onions to side and turn up the heat to high.

Add the ground beef and brown while breaking it apart with a wooden spoon.

Once browned add all the spices, tomato paste and mustard and mix into the meat.

Incorporate the onions into the meat and then add the fresh tomatoes and parsley.

Mix together well and add no more than ¼ cup water to the mix.

Let simmer for 30 minutes or longer (If you can wait to let all the flavors meld together).

While you wait, it's a good time to make the green salad.

The Sunday Roast

Sunday dinner was always eaten at 1pm after church, and it was always a roast of some kind. Here are my two favorite Sunday Roast dinners.

Roast Pork with Apple Sauce

Nothing better than fresh apples in season, so this Sunday Roast was my autumn favorite.

The Pork:

> *6 chop bone-in pork loin roast, about 3lbs*
> *6 whole cloves*
> *Salt and black pepper to taste*

Salt and pepper the roast on all sides.

Make 6 little slits on fat side to insert the cloves, and insert them.

Cook for 90 minutes in a pre-heated 350 degree oven.

Remove, cover with foil and let sit for 20 minutes.

The Apple Sauce:

*4– 6 Fuji or Macintosh apples, peeled
and cored and cut into small pieces.
¼ tsp cinnamon
1/8 tsp each of nutmeg and cloves
1 tbsp butter
¼ cup water*

Put apples and all spices, butter and water in saucepan, set to simmer for about ½ hour.

Mash or use an emersion wand on the softened apples and keep warm until dinner time.

Serve dinner with a great autumn vegetable like Brussels sprouts.

The Sunday Roast, Part II

Roast Chicken with Whipped Cauliflower

Roast chicken and mashed potatoes is the classic American dinner. I loved to eat the neck and the dog got the liver for a treat. Substitute cauliflower for the potatoes and serve with your favorite green vegetable or carrots.

The Chicken:

4lb chicken (pasture raised is the best, otherwise organic is good too, remove any excess fat under skin)
Herb mix of thyme and sage (fresh is best if you can find it)
Salt and pepper

Dry roast the chicken for a crispy skin by just seasoning it with salt, pepper and the herb mix.

Roast in 400 degree preheated oven for 15 minutes, then lower to 350 degrees for one hour 15 minutes.

Remove, cover with foil and let sit for 15 minutes before carving.

The Cauliflower:

1 head of cauliflower
1 garlic clove - minced
3-6 tbsp butter
Salt and black pepper to taste

Cook the cauliflower in about 2 inches of water until soft.

Drain the water from the pot, add butter, salt, black pepper and garlic clove.

Whip with an emersion wand until smooth.

A Holiday Meal Dressing
(for your holiday bird)

*In my family the holiday season meant great stuffing for the bird.
Thanksgiving was a sausage or ham and Christmas was apple and chestnut.
This recipe combines the two, eliminates the bread, but the taste will make
your guests wonder how this can be part of the perfect human diet!*

Baked Apple, Chestnut
and Sausage Dressing

1 ¼ cups almond meal
1 large fuji apple, peeled, cored and diced
10-12 whole chestnuts
2 large pieces of hot (or sweet if you prefer)
Italian sausage, about ½ lb
1 large onion diced
2-3 celery stalks and leaves chopped
¼ to ½ cup vegetable or chicken broth
2 tbsp chopped parsley
2 tbsp olive oil
Salt and black pepper to your liking

Slit the chestnuts with a sharp knife on the flat side, bake them in a 325
degree preheated oven for about 15 minutes, remove, let cool so that
you can touch them, peel and discard the shells and chop the chestnut
meat into small pieces.

In a large sauté pan, cook the onions and celery in 1 tbsp olive oil over a medium heat for about 3 minutes. Remove from the pan and set aside.

Remove the sausage from their casings and brown in the remaining 1 tbsp olive oil for about 10 minutes, breaking the sausage into small pieces as it cooks.

In a large mixing bowl, combine the onion, celery, parsley, apple, chestnuts and sausage. Mix well.

Add in the salt and pepper and the almond meal. Mix and gradually add the broth one tbsp at a time until the dressing is moist but not too wet.

Transfer the dressing onto a shallow baking dish, spreading the mixture out evenly.

Bake in a 350 degree oven for about 1 hour. The top should be golden brown with a slight crisp.

Serve with your holiday bird and other Human Food side dishes for a feast that is perfect.

Next Day Shepherd's Pie

A better way to eat leftovers is to make them into a whole new meal, not just reheated. My mom was a single working parent so she always had to find new and creative ways to make dinner interesting. Here's one:

Reheat the leftover beef stew or shredded pot roast in a pot, and reheat the leftover cauliflower mash (or make new).

Spoon the warmed meat mixture into single serving au gratin dishes or oven tempered bowls, cover with the mash.

Place under the broiler for a few minutes to brown the top of the mash.

Chili Dog

Now that you have all that extra chili, you can make a chili-dog the next day for lunch.

Reheat some chili in a small pot.

Cook your favorite hot-dog but make sure you check the label for additives you don't need or want.

Take a couple of crisp iceberg lettuce leaves instead of a bun. Add your dog and chili on top of the lettuce leaf.

Egg Crepes Sweet or Savory

(who needs pancakes)

I found a great crepe pan in one of those national kitchen stores that make you feel that your kitchen utensils are inadequate, but the special pan makes this recipe easy and possible for everyone to do. This satisfies me when I crave Sunday pancakes that were customary in our house.

4 eggs beaten
Leftover Chili (savory)
Fresh blueberries (sweet)
Salt & white pepper to taste

Melt butter in the pan.

Pour in 2 oz of the egg and swirl around to cover the pan.

Add some reheated chili (savory) or room temperature fresh blueberries (sweet) down the middle of the crepe.

Fold over one side of the egg crepe, then the other side, flip over and slide off into your dish.

Cauliflower Patties

I used to love potato pancakes as a leftover use for the extra mash potatoes. Here is a great substitute for that fondly remembered comfort food.

1 small head of cauliflower
½ medium onion
2/3 cup of blanched almond flour
Salt and black pepper
Olive oil

Rough grate one small head of cauliflower; the head, not the stems.

Rough grate half a medium onion - let it drain and press out excess moisture with paper towel.

Mix the cauliflower and onion together, salt and pepper to taste.

Add 2/3 cup blanched almond flour to the cauliflower-onion mix and incorporate thoroughly.

Beat one medium egg, add to the mixture and mix well.

Heat one large frying pan and add ¼ cup olive oil.

Using a large tablespoon, scoop out some of the cauliflower mixture, place in the palm of hand, and press into a patty.

Place patty into heated oil and brown on a medium heat for a minute to a minute and a half on each side.

Next Day Classic Chicken Soup

Chicken Soup is one of the best one-pot meals you can make. Good when you are sick and great when you are not. Whether you grew up eating it with noodles or rice, just try it this way - pure, simple, and perfectly human. I like soups that are a meal in itself - eat this with our seeded flat bread.

Leftover Roast Chicken carcass with lots of meat left on the bones
4 medium carrots
4 stalks of celery and their leaves
2 small onions
¼ cup roughly chopped parsley
2 tbsp olive oil
Water
Salt and black pepper

Chop your carrots, celery and onion into bite sized pieces.

Heat olive oil in a stockpot; gently cook the chopped vegetables for about 5 minutes.

Season with salt and black pepper, add the parsley.

Add the chicken carcass to the vegetables, then cover the carcass only ¾ of the way with water – too much water and the broth tends to be less rich tasting.

Cover and let simmer for about 2 hours.

Gently remove the carcass from the broth and let cool so that you can remove all the meat.

Add back the meat and bring up to temp.

All American Apple Pie (almost)

Apple pie is the classic American dessert, but it seems that we have been adding so much extra sugar to something that is naturally sweet. That extra sugar plus the refined flour piecrust just wont do. So here is a way of getting that comfort food onto your dessert table once again. This version is a tart so no top crust is needed.

1 1/3 cup blanched almond flour

1 egg beaten

½ tsp salt

1 tbsp softened butter (room temp)

4 small Macintosh apples (if you like a tart taste), or 2 large Gala or Fuji Apples (sweeter)

1 tsp cinnamon

¼ tsp nutmeg

¼ cup water

Mix almond flour, butter salt and egg together to form the dough. Check the moisture content, as you may need to add a bit more butter or flour to get the dough-like consistency.

Refrigerate to cool down while you prepare the apples.

Peel, core, and quarter the apples, then run through your food processor blade.

In a large bowl mix apples with the spices and water to make sure all the apples get coated.

Transfer the apple mixture to a pot and cook on the stovetop over a med heat for about 10-15 minutes. The apples should be slightly softened but not totally limp.

While the apples are simmering, remove dough from the refrigerator and roll out and place into a buttered 8" tart pan. (I line the bottom with parchment paper for easy removal.)

Press the dough into the pan and cook the crust for 5 minutes alone.

Remove the pan from the oven and arrange the partially cooked apple mixture into the tart pan. Dab some butter on top.

Bake in a 325-degree oven for 45-60 minutes or until the crust gets golden brown.

Let the tart cool in the pan for about 15 minutes then pop out the bottom and side the tart onto your favorite serving plate.

Pumpkin Bread

In my family, certain foods only were prepared for the holidays; Pumpkin Pie was one of them (I guess that was because all the pumpkins came into season then).

This guest recipe, courtesy of the Price-Pottenger Nutrition Foundation in San Diego, California, gives us a wonderful alternative to a classic holiday dessert[56].

1/2 cup canned organic pumpkin, or from
fresh organic pumpkin you've cooked yourself.
Eight eggs (organic, free-range or pasture raised)
1/2 cup coconut oil or butter, melted
1/2 cup yacon syrup
1 tsp vanilla (not imitation)
1 1/2 tsp ground cinnamon
1/2 tsp ground mace
1/2 tsp sea salt
3/4 cups sifted coconut flour
1 tsp baking powder
1/2 cup pecans or walnuts, chopped

Blend together pumpkin, eggs, oil, Yacon syrup, vanilla, cinnamon, mace, and salt.

Combine coconut flour with baking powder and whisk thoroughly into batter until there are no lumps.

---

56 This recipe is from *Cooking with Coconut Flower: A Delicious Low-Carb, Gluten-Free Alternative to Wheat* by Bruce Fife, ND (with PPNF's minor alteration of the sweetener). Available from *Price-Pottenger Nutrition Foundation*, www.PPNF.org

Fold in nuts.

Pour into greased 9 x 5 x 3" loaf pan and bake at 350 degrees for 60 minutes.

Remove from pan and cool on rack.

A Final
REPORTER'S NOTE

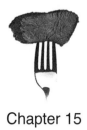

A FINAL
REPORTERS NOTE
THE HEALTH AND
LIFE YOU DESERVE

Chapter 15

"I hope my search will empower you to take control of your own health
where you can, creating the health and life you deserve."

—**CJ Hunt**, in a morning show interview
with a major network affiliate.

N
ow that you understand the concepts and doctor-proven
guidelines behind *The Perfect Human Diet,* you can see how to
put it into practice for the health and life you deserve. I hope
you will take advantage of this authentic method of eating to optimize
your health and wellbeing. By doing that, you will free yourself from
the learned helplessness and failure built into the never-ending supply
of recycled prescriptive diets and diet books. And this is a uniquely
opportune time to do it, when innovative scientific technology is giving
us the answers to questions about the human diet that were previously
unknowable. Answers that clear up the confusion about what foods early

modern humans, humans just like us, were actually eating for well over 100,000 years.

Go for the Gold

When I was competing in the sport of Motocross, an off-road steeplechase on motorcycles, I experienced a community ethic that honored and inspired excellence. Everyone I knew, from beginner class riders to local pros, wanted to be the best they could be. And we looked to the most successful riders in America and Europe, the leaders in the sport, as prime examples of this ethic. Devouring the stories of not only their successes, but the nutrition, physical training, racing skills practice habits, lifestyle and personal commitment they displayed as necessary to compete at the highest levels possible, optimize their results, and achieve their goals. Of course most of what we were learning was new territory, and like all new skills, we expected it to take some time for us to master them and become the best we could be. And in the course of that growth, we all looked to these leaders for inspiration, and they encouraged everyone to rise to the occasion, giving it their all to see just what they could make of themselves.

I'm making a special point of bringing this up because if you search the Internet for diet and health advice, a good number of authors, bloggers and leading personalities will preemptively negate giving it your all. They say you only have to follow their template 80% of the time (or 80% of the way) to get many of the desired results, fearing that the dietary or lifestyle changes will be such a big departure from what you're used to doing that you will bail out after a week or two.

But rather than that approach, I prefer to encourage you to give yourself the gift of reaching as high as possible in order to experience what can happen for you when you give it your all. Respected world-class master trainer Anthony Robbins is well known for telling his audiences how to get the best out of every area of life. It's always a positive message of stretching yourself to new heights and modeling success. One of my favorite quotes of his encourages taking "massive action" to get "massive results." Of course Dr. Sebring, being in the Texas hill country, and not one to mince words, puts it this way, *"Half efforts don't get full results."* It's also more likely that if you aim for 100%, if you happen to fall short of *your* intended goal, that place will still be much higher than aiming low from the start.

The Perfect Human Diet's *Human Food and Non-Human Food*

Several people have mentioned that it helps them to think of these two distinctions, Human Food and Non-Human Food, as their new "rules" of the road. Thinking of these lists as rules helps them use the food lists in a way that effectively guides their choices, therefore attaining, as described in Chapter 3, unconscious competence, easier. Like recognizing the rules of gravity when you're on a the edge of a shear cliff, or drinking clear pure water vs. polluted water, or wanting to breath clean fresh air over smog, these are "rules" that clearly define successful choices.

In addition, we all deserve a trusted source to draw a hard line in the sand when it comes to our health. Watered down concepts and food lists to sell more books or to get more followers will not benefit any of us. With *The Perfect Human Diet,* you now have a clear, doctor proven solution, with vetted lists of what is, or is not, Human Food.

Common Nutrition Ideas that are Wrong (and why)

In a recent interview by *Glamour* magazine Brazil, I was asked to share these new discoveries with their readers in a slightly different way. The magazine wanted me to create a list of five common nutrition ideas that are wrong, based on the hard science discoveries in the film, not my personal opinion. I found it an interesting way to look at the science and wanted to share the *Glamour* magazine list with you.

1. **Meat is Bad:** it's what nature designed us to thrive on.
2. **Animal Fats are Bad**: critical to our developing big brains and current health.
3. **Grains are Healthy**: grains cause inflammation, bind up nutrients, and contribute to much modern disease.

4. **Beans, Grains and Potatoes can replace Animal Foods**: like grains, these are not human foods, negatively impacting our health.

5. **An Optimal Diet is "plant-based"**: animal proteins and fats are irreplaceable in human health.

That's a Wrap!

My search for the solution to obesity and related chronic disease turned out to be an incredibly fascinating treasure hunt. A search that revealed never before seen facts about the authentic human diet and how the well-intentioned inventiveness of our species diverted us from eating Human Food, to novel Non-Human food that is completely out of sync with what our bodies really need for optimal health. It brought to light that we are consuming over 72% of our current diet as Non-Human food, with many authorities insisting we should all continue eating those foods, while at the same time expecting a different health outcome. And it gave us the facts we need to eat in the way that will give us the health and life we deserve.

For the public arena, we now have the knowledge with which to elevate the conversation about what a "healthy diet" really is. And if heeded, stop our downward spiral of increasing obesity and diet related chronic disease, ending the epidemic once and for all.

While there is certain to be those who disagree with these new discoveries, I am hopeful that given the urgency to solve the epidemic most people will be more curious than reactive, more open than defensive. This is *new* scientific knowledge. No one holding a different point of view or belief system about diet could have known the whole picture - until now—when the unknowable became knowable.

ABOUT THE AUTHOR

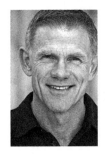

CJ Hunt, filmmaker and broadcast journalist, is the writer, co-executive producer and on camera host of January 2013's #1 Top-Selling Documentary and #1 Top-Selling Independent Film on iTunes, in both the USA and Canada. Mr. Hunt's film also hit #1 Documentary on Amazon Instant Video and Amazon Prime, while making the Top 10 List of All Movies iTunes alongside the major Hollywood blockbusters in the same year. It premiered to over 78 million homes via major USA and Canadian cable systems. As an ongoing audience favorite, the film is now available subtitled in five languages worldwide on multiple platforms.

This book, and his investigative documentary *The Perfect Human Diet*, evolved from his true-life story, beginning in 1978 when paramedics brought Mr. Hunt back to life at the age of 24 after suffering a full cardiac arrest while jogging. That incident evoked an intense passion to find out how we can all achieve longer, healthier and happier lives and then share that information with others.

With over twenty years in broadcasting, voiceovers, television and live events, Mr. Hunt currently lives in Southern California, and is the author of two previous books on diet and health

ACKNOWLEDGEMENTS

This companion book wouldn't exist if it wasn't for the enthusiastic participation of many of the world's top scientists, researchers, and physicians in the evolving field of human evolutionary nutrition who were kind enough to allow me to interview them for my investigative documentary, *The Perfect Human Diet*. I can't thank them enough for giving their time and expertise.

A very special thanks to the *American Museum of Natural History* in New York for opening up their doors and allowing me to film on location in their new Spitzer Hall of Human Origins. The museum is truly amazing, and I highly recommend taking the time to visit when you are in New York.

A big thank you to Morgan James Publishing, New York, for having the faith and vision to support an atypical approach to the diet book genre.

Editor Leslie Farrell whose fine eye and masterful clarifications are always much appreciated.

And finally, to my friend, Ray Grant, for his 24/7 support and word processor savvy that has helped me leap over the many manuscript-formatting hurdles in time to make my deadlines.

RESOURCES

www.CJHuntReports.com
For the most current resources, news and information you are invited to CJ's website and blog.

Free Bonus Book Extras
www.ThePerfectHumanDietBook.com/extras

Suggested Supplements
Carlson Lemon Flavored Cod Liver Oil (not the unflavored)
Perfect Family by SuperNutrition (Multivitamin)
Jarro-Dophilus +FOS by Jarrow Formulas (Acidophilus)

Press, Speaking, Screenings and Business Inquiries
Contact George Thompson, Managing Partner
GThompson@HuntThompsonMedia.com

ABOUT THE #1 DOCUMENTARY

To view the trailer for *The Perfect Human Diet* and learn more about where you can see, purchase or rent it, please visit my new website www.CJHuntReports.com

Film Synopsis

The Perfect Human Diet is the unprecedented global exploration for a solution to our epidemic of overweight, obesity and diet-related diseases - the #1 killer in America. This film, by broadcast journalist C.J. Hunt, bypasses current dietary group-think by exploring modern dietary science, previous historical findings, ancestral native diets and the emerging field of human dietary evolution - revealing for the first time, the authentic human diet. Film audiences finally can see what our species truly needs for optimal health and are given a practical template based on scientific facts.

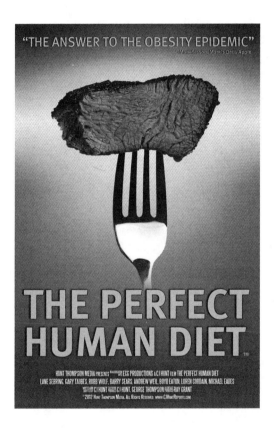

Film Cast

C.J. Hunt
Lane Sebring, M.D.
Robb Wolf
Gary Taubes
Loren Cordain, PhD
Michael R. Eades, M.D.
Jay Wortman, M.D.
David Getoff, CCN
Barry Sears, PhD
Gary J. Sawyer
Leslie Aiello, PhD
Jean Jacque Hublan, PhD
Mike Richards, PhD
Shannon McPherron, PhD
Maria Soressi, PhD
Andrew Weil, M.D.
Boyd Eaton, M.D.
Adele Hilte, MPH. MAT.
Sally Fallon Morrell, MA
Joel Fuhrman, M.D.
Alan Goldhamer, D.C.

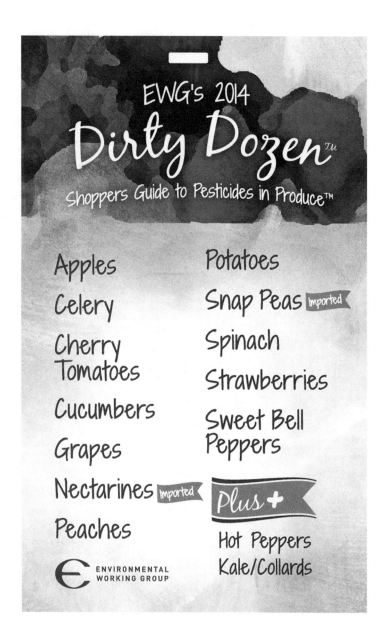

EWG's 2014

Clean Fifteen™

Shoppers Guide to Pesticides in Produce™

Asparagus	Mangoes
Avocados	Onions
Cabbage	Papayas
Cantaloupe	Pineapples
Cauliflower	Sweet Corn
Eggplant	Sweet Peas Frozen
Grapefruit	Sweet Potatoes
Kiwi